Department of Health

Care Staff in Transition

The impact on staff of changing services
for people with mental handicaps

PETER ALLEN, JAN PAHL, LYN QUINE

LONDON: HMSO

Acknowledgements

This book is based on research which was funded by the (then) Department of Health and Social Security and we are grateful for the support that we received. However, the views expressed in this book are the responsibility of the authors and do not necessarily represent the official views of the Department.

We should like to thank all those people who gave their time and advice to us during the research: these include the members of the Steering Group who diligently criticised our plans, the management and staff of the pilot hospital who helped us improve our questionnaire and Barbara Holland and Linda McDonnell who patiently typed and retyped our manuscript.

Our thanks also go to the residents who welcomed us into their homes during the course of our research. Our greatest debt is to those members of staff who completed our long questionnaire and who readily gave of their time to help us understand the problems being faced in this time of great change.

Peter Allen
Jan Pahl
Lyn Quine

The Authors

Peter Allen (BSc, PhD) is joint head of Psychology at the Robens Institute of Health and Safety, University of Surrey.

Jan Pahl (MA, PhD) is Director of Research at the National Institute for Social Work.

Lyn Quine (BA, PhD) is Senior Research Fellow at the Institute of Social and Applied Psychology, University of Kent.

Contents

List of Tables and Figures

1 Introduction

This book is about staff working in two organisations which provide care for people with mental handicaps. It is based on the results of an intensive study of staff characteristics and experience which was intended to provide general lessons for those providing such services. The two organisations were an NHS long-stay hospital, which was subject to a closure programme, and a new local authority staffed housing service which was receiving some of the residents from the hospital and employing a number of its ex-staff.

During the period in which we conducted this research, Sir Roy Griffiths was undertaking an overview of community care policy with the aim of providing guidance for action in this complex and changing area (Griffiths, 1988). As we shall outline in the next chapter, there has been a gradual increase in the services provided in the community by local authorities and a continuing reduction in long-stay hospital services based in NHS hospitals. The Griffiths review endorsed this general trend and recommended that local authorities should have major responsibility for community care. In 1989 (just as this book goes to print) the Government published its White Paper on Community Care, which made it clear that the main Griffith recommendations had been accepted, thus the trend of hospital closure and local community care development should continue and grow (Secretaries of State for Health, 1989).

The difficulties concerning staff transferring from NHS hospitals to local authority services constitute one particular problem which was noted in the Griffiths review (para. 6.15). But the development of local community services, and even the possible transfer of responsibility for some NHS services to local authorities, raises many issues relating to staff. Bearing in mind the historical trend it is clear that the whole thrust of development is towards a re-definition of the job as well as towards a change of setting (Brown and Walton, 1984 p.10). How are staff to be recruited and selected for the new community services? Will they be drawn from the hospital sector or from other parts of the labour market? Will skills and attitudes developed in hospitals still be relevant in the new community services? What can be done to retain staff as hospitals decline in size?

Allied to these concerns are questions about training. What are the training needs of those working in the new service? Are there additional training requirements in the hospital that are linked in some way to the decline in resident numbers? How do the changes affect staff morale and confidence? How do staff respond to the different structures and demands of the two services? Are their reactions more or less similar or are they different in kind?

In order to address these questions, we needed to make some minimum assumptions about staff reactions. Although staff could be expected to identify specific problems which they had encountered, the severity of effect of any sort of problem, be it a pattern of working, an organisational feature or the degree of client handicap, would be difficult to measure. Thus we planned the study on the assumption that whatever arrangements are made, or changes initiated in the services, any non-trivial problems which are generated for staff will appear in measures of job satisfaction, in propensity to leave and as more general indications of work related stress.

This is essentially an applied social psychological perspective and matches that of Kahn et al. (1964) which viewed stress as the reaction of employees to those aspects of the work situation which they perceived as threatening. In this model stress is likely to be the result of a mis-match between individuals' abilities and the requirements of their work. Stress will occur either when excessive demands are made of employees or when employees are inadequately equipped to cope with a situation. In applying this approach we intended to provide some indication of the relative weight to be given to those aspects of the work situation which staff identified as problematic.

Similarly by including measures of job satisfaction, we hoped to identify the major dimensions of the work responsible for reducing rewards in either or both settings. By including both stress and satisfaction measures in an analysis of 'propensity to leave' we could also trace some of those features of the work which were leading to increased turnover. Both job dissatisfaction (Johnson and Stinson, 1975; Lyons, 1971; Miles, 1975) and turnover (Gupta and Beehr, 1979) have been linked to stress, but there is no agreed general model for the exact nature of such links (Jamal, 1984). Since our aims did not require the testing of a specific or detailed model of this type we could treat these measures as indicators of the relative importance of those job factors which differed between the two types of service.

Our overall strategy, therefore, was to measure those kinds of outcomes for staff which might derive from the features of the job and then to explore the attributed causes and occurrence of problems in each setting. The focus was on those aspects of the situation which could be identified as having their roots in the move to the community.

This strategy called for at least two types of information: well defined measures of work outcomes together with their most likely correlates, and more discursive accounts of work patterns and of the problems encountered by care staff. Given the largely cross-sectional nature of the research, and the kinds of issues involved, the obvious framework was comparative, distinguishing between staff in the two settings but using identical measures, at least for the outcomes and related variables.

The study fell into two main phases and involved three kinds of methods; these were unstructured observation, a postal survey with a standardised instrument, and extended interviewing with a simple random sample of staff drawn from the hospital and all the staff from the community, and with management of the two organisations. The latter included the director of nursing services, assistant director and unit general manager at the hospital, and the director and officers of the community service.

At the design stage it was not clear what information we would be able to obtain about the turnover of those staff who completed our questionnaire. In fact during the second phase we were able to check back from the hospital employment records, because we had identified each questionnaire with a code number in order that reminder letters could be sent out during the postal survey, and this provided us with an extremely valuable longitudinal element to the research. Equally it was not clear to what extent we could analyse responses within the hospital by villa or unit. In the event the fluidity of the situation during the period of the research, and the operating procedures of the hospital, made this an unprofitable line to pursue.

The design of the postal questionnaire depended on our need to cover the full range of likely influences on staff outcomes, as well as those outcomes themselves. The final version of the questionnaire, which is reproduced as an Appendix, contained four main types of question: staff demographics, job perceptions, work attitudes and responses to the job. Only the first of these types used open format questions. Explanations of the measures based on these questions appear in the appropriate sections of the book.

The postal questionnaires were distributed to all the direct care staff at the hospital and in the community service using those organisations' internal mail systems. Questionnaires were returned direct to the research team by pre-paid post. We received a total of 271 completed usable questionnaires, which represented 58 per cent of the total number of staff. Twenty-seven of these were from the community (87 per cent response rate) and 244 from the hospital (56 per cent). This was a reasonable response for such a survey, given that the questionnaire contained 157 individual items within its 14 pages.

There was also a fairly uniform response with respect to the different groups within the organisations. Of the four community service officers three replied. All five managers of staffed houses responded and the 19 community basic care staff who replied represented 86 per cent of that grade. The response rates of the different hospital groups are shown below:

3

	N	(Per cent)
Directors and nursing officers	11	92
Charge nurses and sisters	34	59
Registered nurses	26	59
Enrolled nurses	32	42
Nursing assistants	121	50
Therapists and others	20	40

The only major difference in these rates concerns nursing officers, nearly all of whom replied.

The interview schedule was designed after the preliminary analysis of the results obtained from the postal survey. It was intended to cover much the same ground as the questionnaire but in a qualitatively different manner. Topics were identified on the schedule in the same basic order as on the questionnaire but the interviewee was able to talk about the topics in as natural a fashion as possible. Each topic was checked off as it occurred in the conversation, points of interest were followed up and additional clarification sought as necessary. Cues, derived from the questionnaire analysis, were included on the schedule. We completed 62 intensive interviews with care staff, which represents an 86 per cent overall response rate from our sample. These interviews took a considerable time to complete, rarely less than an hour and a half and often more than two hours. We were struck by the response of basic care staff who often remarked that they and their views had been ignored for too long. Our interviews with the managers were also very detailed and we were consequently able to relate our findings from the questionnaire and the care staff interviews to the details of policy implementation, as these were perceived by those in charge.

A note on presentation

Although the data were collected in these two separate phases, they are combined by topic in this book which is structured around the main issues. Because most of the scales in the questionnaire were of the Likert type (see Ghiselli et al., 1981) the actual numerical values used on each scale are arbitrary and we have therefore minimised the reporting of results using those values in order not to overburden the text with numbers that have meaning only within the context of a given scale. Instead we have presented many results as bar charts where the length of a bar represents the (standardised) score of a particular group in terms of how much more, or less, it is than the overall average for that measure.

For similar reasons the interview responses are only reported as percentages. Usually these percentages were calculated for the whole sample, but in some cases they are the proportions of a set of responses. We have labelled these tables accordingly. By convention all percentages are calculated by each column within a table.

Finally, and in order to improve readability throughout the book, we have avoided including too many details of statistical analyses. Where we refer to differences or effects, the reader should assume that those differences are large enough to be genuine rather than chance fluctuations. We have tested all such differences and effects using appropriate inductive techniques and usually report the level of probability used to judge the likelihood involved. Where differences fall below this level we have usually described them as due to chance. Thus a value reported as $(p < .05)$ means that the reported difference (or other type of effect) would only be found in a large number of similar surveys less than once every 20 times. A smaller value for 'p' of course means that the reported difference is even less likely to be due to chance. Details of the scales and their statistical characteristics are given in Appendix I.

2 Setting the Scene

This chapter describes the context of the study which is the basis of this book. We begin with a brief review of the evolution of policy on community care and then go on to describe the ways in which the various English Regions have changed their service provision. Finally we describe the long-stay hospital and the new local authority community service which employed the staff who were the main subjects of our research.

Community care

At the time of writing community care has become something of a confusing term (Malin, 1987; House of Commons, 1985, Vol. 1 para. 8). Twenty years ago a series of studies and scandals focussed attention on large scale institutions and the long term care which they provided (Tizard, 1964; Morris, 1969; DHSS, 1969; King et al., 1971). At that time community care, though ill-defined, tended to imply a service that was not provided in a large hospital. Subsequently there has been considerable development in the breadth of meaning of this phrase, and a dramatic impact on the nature of the services providing care.

There has also been a continued development of national policy. The 1971 White Paper (DHSS, 1971) 'Better Services for the Mentally Handicapped' recommended that local authority establishments should be used for those people who did not have physical handicaps or behavioural problems requiring special medical or nursing skills (para. 158). A year later the Briggs Committee on Nursing (1972) recommended movement towards 'a realignment in care of the mentally handicapped between health and social services' (p.172), and proposed that training of nurses in the field of mental handicap should place more emphasis 'on the social aspects of care' (recommendation 74, p.217). The recommendations included reference to the gradual emergence of a 'new caring profession' but it was unclear what the further implications of such a development might be. In order to examine the 'care of the mentally handicapped in the light of developing policies', a committee of enquiry was set up which reported in 1979 (Jay Report, p.1). The 1971 White Paper had suggested that local authority places should expand by six times and that one half of hospital places should go, but the whole emphasis of the Jay Report was determined by a 'Model of Care' based on a set of principles which the committee described as their philosophy. The implications for services were that 'specialised' services or organisations should be just that, providing for additional needs rather than providing the bulk of basic care. The favoured environment was to consist of 'adapted houses which are physically integrated with the community' (p.35). Three broad sets of principles were elaborated.

(a) Mentally handicapped people have a right to enjoy normal patterns of life within the community.
(b) Mentally handicapped people have a right to be treated as individuals.
(c) Mentally handicapped people will require additional help from the communities in which they live and from professional services if they are to develop to their maximum potential as individuals (para. 89).

The committee went some way in turning these principles into recommendations for practice. Its emphasis on 'normal patterns of life' reflected contemporary international thinking on philosophies of care (UN Declaration of the Rights of Mentally Handicapped Persons, 1972; Wolfensberger, 1972; and see Tyne and O'Brien, 1981).

In 1980 the DHSS published its review of progress in services for mentally handicapped people (DHSS, 1980). Its conclusions included the idea that targets for hospital places for children and adults were probably too high (paras. 2.39; 2.47). It further encouraged a joint approach between health and social services and the voluntary sector. Whereas the 1971 White Paper had seen a future need for 200-bed, district-based units for adults, the review considered that few districts would need more than 150 health care places – and those not necessarily on the same site. The push towards community based services was given more impetus in 1981 by the consultative document 'Care in the Community' (DHSS, 1981). It estimated that 'about 15,000 mentally handicapped people at present in hospital could be discharged immediately if appropriate services in the community were available' (para. 3.1). This figure represented approximately a third of the then in-patient numbers. The principle of community based care was re-affirmed (para. 1.1) by the statement that those needing long-term care 'should be looked after in the community'. In 1983 a circular setting out the altered principles for the transfer of joint finance to local authorities was published (DHSS, 1983). Health authorities could then transfer funding to local authorities or voluntary organisations to set up schemes to care for people who would otherwise need hospital places.

In 1985, the year in which this research began, the Second Report from the Social Services Committee Session (House of Commons, 1985) recommended that in the long term all social care mental handicap facilities should be supported by local authorities. For most adults this would be in the form of ordinary housing within the community. The report showed that expenditure on residential care for people with mental handicaps had increased five times more than the average increase on all social services spending between 1975 and 1981. The historical trend therefore was to reduce hospital provision.

In 1986 Sir Roy Griffiths was commissioned to review the policy of community care. He was asked to produce a brief review geared to advice on action, and duly reported in 1988. In his call for the clarification of the responsibilities of health authorities he noted that:

> It has been Government policy for many years that long stay hospitals for mentally ill, mentally handicapped and elderly people are not, in general, the right setting for people who do not need both medical supervision and nursing care to be available throughout 24 hours, although there will be a continuing need for some long stay hospital facilities....

His recommendations were 'intended to enable that policy to be implemented more effectively', (para. 4.13).

Thus the historical trend outlined above should continue and regional health authorities should make 'specific plans ... for the reduction in long stay hospital beds' (para. 6.37). Responsibility for community care should, in general, fall to local authorities.

Regional variations

How had this well established trend in policy been translated into service provision up to the period of our research? To set our study into its national context there were two questions to be asked about current service provision: what kinds of changes had so far taken place and at what rate had the relevant changes occurred? Approximately coincident with the start of this research many District and Regional Health Authorities published their strategy documents for the 10 year period to 1994. These enabled us to outline the beginnings of some answers to our two questions, whilst published Departmental statistics helped by providing some standard comparative figures. Although these strategies were drawn up before the present Government accepted the recommendations made by Sir Roy Griffiths the variations they revealed reflect deep seated differences which, whatever the detail of future policy, will probably still have visible consequences for many years to come.

Indeed the most noticeable feature of current service provision is its diversity; there are a number of different types of service and within each there is a considerable further variation. It was not surprising therefore, to find that the regional strategy documents also varied in their approach. The overall trend was in line with the policy recommendations we have briefly summarized but interpretation into changes in services varied widely. Most regions based their future provision on some version of the philosophy set out in the Jay Report, but two regions began their discussion of services without any explicit philosophy and two spoke only of reductions in hospital based services, or of NHS provision being for short term care. Most regions, however, proposed to reduce in-patient numbers in their various hospitals. The range of projected reductions in long-stay institutional care was enormous. The lowest estimated total reduction in the period to 1994 was 11 per cent, the highest 100 per cent. Two regions did not set figures to their hospital reductions but on all the available estimates, there seemed likely to be an average reduction in in-patient numbers of 59 per cent in England as a whole.

Hospital closures were a prime target for the strategic period. If we included those described as possible closures within the period then the total of large hospitals (>100 beds) projected to close was 16. In addition some 30 smaller hospitals were listed as likely to close or planned to close. From 1979 to 1985, 13 hospitals had been approved for closure in England and nine of those had actually closed by 1984 (Wertheimer, 1986). It is the overall reduction in the numbers of in-patients, however, rather than hospital closures, that is the main feature of mental handicap services both in the past two decades and in the planned period to 1994. Although only two regions avoided any mention of hospital closures, all regions recognised the likelihood of reductions in the numbers of long-stay patients.

There are three main reasons for the decline in the total population in hospitals:

(i)   The numbers of new long-stay patients have reduced (partly because new admissions are not accepted).
(ii)   Older patients have died.
(iii)   New residential facilities have received discharged long stay patients.

Again there is considerable variation in the rate of loss within each region. In the nine years from 1977 to 1985 the range of reduction was from 17.8 per cent to 30.9 per cent, an average reduction of 23.8 per cent. One related consequence of a larger rate of reduction in many regions was a rise in the proportion of long-stay residents. In some regions the proportion of the total hospital population who had been resident for five years or more was larger than nine years before, in others it was smaller. In 1985, the range of the proportion of 'long-stay' as opposed to 'short-term care' patients was considerable, varying from 68.1 per cent to 91.7 per cent, an average of 81.5 per cent in the English Regions as a whole.

Discharging a considerable proportion of all residents while decreasing the proportion of longer-stay residents implies that a 'change of use' philosophy is being pursued, for example, where facilities are more often being used to provide short-term respite care. On the other hand a high rate of discharge and an *increase* in the proportion of long-stay residents implies a concentration of people who are less readily placed in the community (Jones, 1975, p.96). Figure 2.1 plots two measures of changes in the structure of regional long-stay facilities in order to identify such variations in the practices of the 14 regions.

Of course other interpretations for what is actually happening can be made using the data, but the experience of those in the mental handicap field seems to accord quite well with the differences this simple plot reveals. The vertical axis in Figure 2.1 records the percentage reduction in the total number of in-patients during the period to 1985 (based on 1977) and the horizontal axis records the change in the proportion of long stay residents between 1977 and 1985. The broken lines represent the average values on each scale. Thus regions above the horizontal broken line lost more than the average proportion of residents of all kinds, and regions to the left of the vertical broken line either reduced the proportion of long stay residents,

Figure 2.1

Regional variations in the reduction of the proportion of long-stay residents and the relative composition of hospital populations for 1977 to 1985

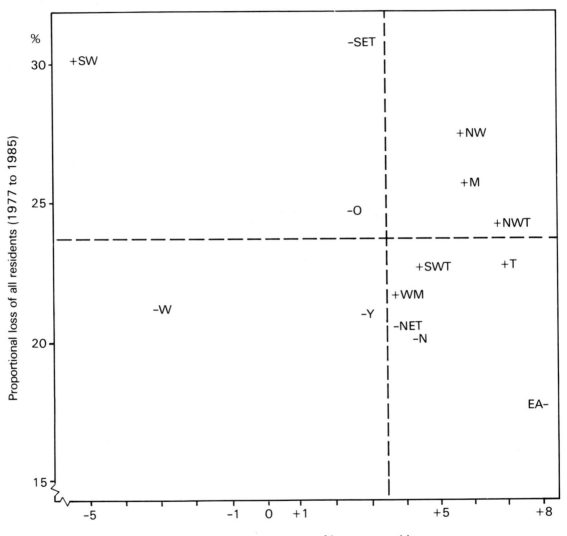

Key
N: Northern; Y: Yorkshire; T: Trent; EA: East Anglian; NWT: North West Thames;
NET: North East Thames; SET: South East Thames; SWT: South West Thames; W: Wessex;
O: Oxford; SW: South Western; WM: West Midlands; M: Mersey; NW: North Western.

'+' Above average size region; '-' Below average size region.

Source: DHSS 1974 to 1987

or increased it by a less than average amount. Notice that the average change was in fact an *increase* in the proportion of long-stay residents.

Added to the identifying symbols in Figure 2.1 are plus and minus signs: these indicate regions that have a larger (+) or smaller (−) number of mentally handicapped hospital residents than average (usually due to the siting of large long-stay hospitals). Note that all but one of the larger regions increased the proportion of long-stay residents during the period. The original proportions of long-stay residents were greater in the larger regions. In other words the size of the region was related to the proportion of long stay residents; the larger the region the greater the proportion of long-stay residents. Since 1977, most large regions have increased that proportion still further.

What of the long term trend? How have in-patient numbers changed during the period covered by the policy documents we have discussed? Has the rate of change been constant, or is there increasing activity? A useful summary of these trends is given by Taylor and Taylor (1986). In 1970 there were 55,434 people estimated to be in-patients in NHS hospitals and units. Apart from an erratic shift following the White Paper in 1971, this number has fallen and has done so at an increasing rate. There was a noticeable upturn in 1983–84 following publication of the circular which clarified the principles for joint finance arrangements (DHSS, 1983). If we extrapolate from this trend then, at the time of writing, the annual rate of reduction is probably about 7 per cent.

As the numbers of hospital residents have declined the provision of places in local authority control has risen. Between 1970 and 1985 there was a 217 per cent increase in such places to a total of 15,152. DHSS statistics show both staffed and unstaffed homes. There have been dramatic changes in the yearly rate of growth of both types of provision. One way to show the size of this growth is to compare it directly with the contemporary hospital provision. In 1970 the number of local authority places represented 7.9 per cent of the total provision, that is of hospital and local authority provision combined, while in 1985 this proportion had risen to 29.4 per cent. The number of places in unstaffed homes has grown more rapidly over the period (1975–85) at an average rate of 16 per cent per year, compared to the growth of places in staffed homes at 4.8 per cent per year. However, the bulk of provision is in staffed homes, which provide nearly eight times as many places as unstaffed houses.

Part of the reason for this difference in scale relates to the average size of 'homes'. The staffed units are more likely to be hostels and they have an average of nearly five times as many residents as the unstaffed. However, a further minor trend can be discerned in the official figures. Since 1975 the average number of places per local authority unit has declined, for both staffed and unstaffed units. In 1975 the average size of a staffed unit was 20.8 people and this gradually decreased each year to 19.4 in 1985. Similarly the average size of unstaffed units was 4.9 people in 1975 and this had decreased to 4.1 by 1985. Thus there has been both an increase in local authority provision and a decrease in the size of local authority units although, as these figures indicate, the physical provision remains mostly of the hostel rather than the house. (Anderson, 1982, Malin et al., 1980).

Part of the driving force for this reduction in the scale of units has been the pursuit of the new philosophies of care discussed above. The emphasis on 'normal patterns of life' has often been taken to imply limits to the acceptable maximum scale of individual units, as well as their geographical location. At the same time the findings of the research conducted in the 1960s and 1970s have led to attempts to change the nature of staff-client interactions, which were found to be enhanced by a smaller scale.

One of the major implications of all these changes is an increasing demand for staff to operate the growing number of local authority units. At the same time NHS staff requirements are unlikely to shrink and may even grow. Regional manpower estimates vary, with a majority of strategic documents giving no firm figure for staffing, but anything up to 48.5 per cent growth is envisaged by those few regions giving figures. Many of the developments which are proposed will grow out of existing NHS provision. For example, most regions have, and plan to increase, Community Mental Handicap Teams. These also vary greatly in their composition, size and in the nature of their work (Plank, 1982). Some NHS units may remain to become the specialised core in a 'core and cluster' model of otherwise 'ordinary' houses or units (King's Fund, 1980). Community placement continues to grow with 'Adult Fostering' arrangements and voluntary and private provision. Some health districts, following earlier policy directions, have already placed long-term residents in new 200 bed units. In contrast the small units favoured in some regions, are recommended to be always less than 25 residents and preferably less than 16 (eg Oxford RHA, 1984). As we have suggested, however, there appears to be a long term trend to reduce the size of community units and this would seem especially likely to continue, given the new post-Griffiths initiative for the role of local authorities.

Thus our research is concerned with two situations which are pertinent to current provision and likely future developments: the reduction and closure of a large NHS hospital and the development of a local authority staffed housing service based on ordinary houses in the community.

The local hospital

The hospital was originally the smaller of two large mental handicap hospitals in the region. The Regional Health Authority (RHA) decided to close the largest of these in 1979, at which time the two hospitals together held nearly two-thirds of all the adult mentally handicapped people in hospital in the region. The closure of the hospital we have studied was decided upon in 1983 and a 10 year closure plan was produced at the end of 1984. By that time the region had reduced its total hospital population by 21.6 per cent and the relative balance between the two main hospitals had changed. The first had shrunk by 34.5 per cent so that it was nearly 15 per cent smaller than the second. The RHA Strategic Plan anticipated closure of the first hospital by 1988.

Our research began in 1985, just over a year after the closure plan appeared. At that time the hospital had over 650 residents, but by 1987 it was down to 530. The reduction in size did not begin with the closure plan announcement: like most large scale units in the country the hospital had been reducing slowly since reaching its maximum of about 1,500 in the 1960s. There was a noticeable increase in the rate of reduction once the closure plan was announced but the relative numbers of residents of different dependency levels changed at different rates. From 1984 to 1987 the hospital lost 48.1 per cent of its low dependency residents and 27.8 per cent of its medium dependency residents but only 23 per cent of its high dependency residents. Obviously, as a result of this concentration process, the proportions of each dependency level within the hospital have changed. By 1987 only 10 per cent of the hospital population were in the low dependency category, while 36 per cent were high dependency.

The hospital itself dates back to 1928 when the main building was converted from a private home for use as a hospital for 'mental defectives'. The additional buildings, the villas, began to be erected in the 1930s and were still being added to in the late 1950s. The hospital occupies a large and very attractive rural site, about one and a half miles from the nearest small town. The villas are spread out in the grounds, and typically, at the time the research began, each housed around 20–30 residents. The villas are grouped according to type and level of handicap in the manner that most accounts in the literature have made familiar (eg Alaszewski, 1986). In addition to the usual layout with dormitory and day room, several villas have been converted into 'flats' and have some domestic facilities. There is also a large house on the perimeter of the site used for community training, a halfway house and a hospital block. There are three training units and three specialist therapy departments. During the period of the research one villa was converted into a special unit for people with severely challenging behaviour.

Under the closure plan the loss of each resident, including those that die, reduces the hospital's revenue budget. The logic of the reduction implies that wards or villas should close as units, enhancing the savings on running costs. Usually this means that when the population of a given villa reduces to a certain minimum the remaining residents are re-distributed to other villas so that the unit may close. When our research began three villas had already closed and three more were closed in that year. In the following year another three were closed and, in the last year (1987) four more villas were closed, to leave 18.

Within its local area the hospital constitutes a fairly major industry. It employs many people in addition to its nursing staff. There were 47 employees in administration, 44 in estate maintenance and 210 in other support services such as the laundry and catering. There were 54 medical/therapy staff. The nursing staff constituted only 56 per cent of the total work force when our research began. The nursing staff establishment had been at around 425 whole time equivalents in the late 1970s and this increased by as much as a quarter during the early 1980s. The largest increases followed the introduction of the $37\frac{1}{2}$ hour week in 1980–81. The closure plan brought in tight budgetary controls and subsequently the number of staff has fallen. The loss has been achieved by reducing recruitment and by transferring staff from closing villas. By 1987 the nursing establishment had returned to its 1970s levels of 430 whole time equivalents. Because the number of residents had fallen consistently throughout this period the nurse/resident ratio has actually improved. In 1983 this ratio was 0.69 and by the time our research began it was already up to 0.78. Our study was confined to the nursing staff, including nursing assistants.

There is a nursing school attached to the hospital which has a total of 72 places, and produces an average of 24 newly qualified nurses per year. Up to, and even beyond, the announcement of the closure programme the supply of newly qualified staff from the school was high. Indeed, there was often a waiting list for new staff posts at the hospital. Subsequently the number of students coming forward has dropped, partly because of funding policy, so that by 1987 the school was down to two thirds of its capacity.

Two other developments have affected the situation. In line with the changes to the training syllabus, introduced by the English National Board in 1982 to re-orientate nurse training towards community care, the school has greatly reduced the time students spend in the hospital: approximately 40 per cent of their time is now spent on the villas. Furthermore, when students qualify they are considerably less likely to apply for posts at the hospital. Applications were down in 1987 to about half the reduced number of qualifying staff. Together these changes have placed a strain on the level of qualified staffing within the hospital.

Leaving rates, the other side of the turnover process, were at a relatively high level for all grades. The full list of care staff with which we were provided at the beginning of the study enabled us to check back on those who were no longer employed after the first year and a half had elapsed. Table 2.1 gives the proportion of staff from each grade who had left. These are adjusted annual equivalent proportions and are calculated using the original staff list as the denominator. There are well known difficulties in the definition of appropriate turnover measures. This is a crude separation rate, such as employed by Mercer (1979). However, since our concern was with comparisons by grade within the hospital, and between hospital and community, the only requirement was that we use one calculating method for both organisations. The overall average rate for the hospital was 17.6 per cent per annum.

The difference between leaving rates for different grades of staff could well be due to chance, however, ($p < .1$) and, generally, the leaving rate for all grades was fairly stable.

Table 2.1
Leaving rates of hospital
staff by grade

Grade	Rate (per cent per annum)
Nursing officers and above	16.7
Villa management (charge nurses and sisters)	13.8
Registered staff nurses	21.2
Enrolled nurses	18.4
Nursing assistants	17.7

Towards the end of the second year of the research, structural changes in the organisation altered the employment opportunities of qualified staff. Under the original administration each villa was managed by a charge nurse and a sister, who worked different shifts, and the villas were organised into five groups under nursing officers. The closure programme reduced the scale of operations and the number of groups had already been reduced. Following the appointment of the Unit General Manager under the new NHS structure, further changes were implemented. The clinical services were placed in charge of one manager, and, at villa level, responsibility was vested in one manager with a deputy. The span of control of the villa managers was extended to 24 hour coverage. Staff had to apply for the new positions, which were advertised.

The new community service

The community service was set up at the beginning of 1984 and the first care staff were appointed later that year. It was set up to develop a community based range of services for people with mental handicaps within the health district. It is important to note that the community service and the hospital were located in different health districts. The community service was operated by the social services department of the local authority but was funded by the health authority. The first development was to be in staffed houses and the first and most significant target group for receipt of the new service were the hospital residents whose original homes had been in the health district.

The regional and district health authorities provided capital funding for the purchase and development of the houses. These were intended to be ordinary houses, not especially large or set apart from any others. Revenue funding for the service was also to be provided by the health authority. An index linked sum, originally £10,300, was to be released to the service with each person who left a long stay NHS unit to return to their district of origin. At the time that the service was set up 197 people were identified as having originally come from the district. In addition some 50 people, whose original district was unknown, were to be catered for by the service. Of the total of 247 potential clients 75 per cent were resident in the hospital that we were to study.

Some of the hospital residents could be discharged to the voluntary and private sector but the rest would be cared for by the service directly. Some would require physically adapted houses; all needed permanent 24 hour care. It was anticipated that some 50 clients could be discharged to families through an adult placement scheme in which carers would continue to receive support from the service. During the hospital closure period a further number of clients, who had been discharged to the staffed houses, were expected to be transferred to this scheme.

From 1985 to 1994 the number of staffed houses was to grow to a total of 29 houses, 17 of which would require physical adaptation. Each house would provide a home for up to four people and would employ a 'house co-ordinator' and some five 'house companions' or basic care staff. The planned growth was for a total of 191 staff by the end of the period.

At an early stage two large properties on the edge of the hospital estate were rented to the community service to act as half-way houses, so that residents and staff could prepare for the full move out to the ordinary houses in their home district. By 1985 the service had discharged 15 hospital residents to its staffed houses, four to their home district and 11 to the two half-way houses. By the end of 1986 four houses were in operation and new residents in both half-way houses were awaiting moves to the two properties that would be ready in 1987. The overall care staff to resident ratio was 1.2 at that time.

The care staff were employed by social services on the residential social worker scale with an additional allowance payable for the 'sleep-in' shift which staff were required to work as necessary. Staff were employed on this scale in order that people with at least some experience of operating in a community setting could be recruited, but it was not intended that this should limit the applicants to the posts. Indeed, there was awareness that no existing qualification exactly matched the nature of the jobs being created. There was an early recognition that, as the service grew and according to the needs of more challenging clients, there would be a need for perhaps 60 per cent of the house co-ordinators to be trained qualified nurses and for other staff to have additional experience and training in behaviour management. There were no limitations on the qualifications for house companions, who were recruited for their 'strong commitment and motivation'.

When data collection began there were three people in the service management team and an attached social worker. There were six house co-ordinators and together with the house companions this made a total of 36 staff. Of these staff four were RNMH, three were SENs and three had social work qualifications. The rest were unqualified but only nine had had no previous experience of working with people with a mental handicap.

There was a clear recognition by the service that people with nursing qualifications would be appropriate employees. Indeed, as the number of clients with greater dependency and special needs increased, there was a policy of seeking to employ qualified nurses. Although the nursing component of the unit was expected to vary with residents' needs there was no policy of excluding nurses from employment in houses where that component

16

was thought to be minimal and nurse training was generally valued. In fact some management experience at least in the sense of preparedness to take responsibility, which many qualified nurses could claim, was also appreciated from the outset.

Recruitment of staff proved to be rather variable during the first years of the service. In order that its staff should be able to relate appropriately to the residents, the aim was to recruit people across the age range and to recruit both men and women, since residents in the houses were of mixed sex. The residents were equally divided between men and women and this implied a need for similarly balanced proportions of male and female staff. There was some success in this. By the end of 1986 about a third of the staff who had been employed, including those who had left, had been men. The rate of leaving the community service was high overall but there was no evidence of a difference between men and women with respect to leaving. During the first 18 months of the research the proportions of male and female community staff who had left were virtually identical (31 and 29 per cent respectively). Achieving and maintaining an equal proportion of male and female staff seemed to turn, therefore, on recruitment rather than on retention.

We noted that the leaving rate for the community service as a whole was high. This is a comparative judgement. The rate, adjusted in the same way as reported for the hospital, was 22.9 per cent per annum. This rate is higher than that for the hospital by an amount that is unlikely to be due to chance ($p < 0.05$) and this is probably because, as we report below, of the rather different compositions of the two work forces. However, rates this high are not uncommon in the field of basic grade social work (Knapp et al., 1981).

Opportunities for advancement within the new service were initially quite limited. Given the development plans, however, the future structure of the service would require an expanded range of intermediate managerial posts. At first the growth of the service was slower than had been anticipated, partly because of the need for change-of-use planning permission by the County Council. The increase in the number of management positions was an early need. Initially the management team mounted the staff induction courses but as the service expanded this became difficult to sustain. By 1986–87 there was a shortfall of managerial support and a community co-ordinator was appointed to manage some of the houses whilst another officer was appointed to manage the property acquisition and other non-professional aspects of the service.

At the same time a grant from the European Social Fund made the appointment of a Staff Development and Training Officer feasible. This post was funded for three years under an arrangement by which the European Social Fund would meet half the cost while the other half would be met from social services and health service sources. The need for an additional training input was apparent once the operational duties of the management team precluded their further contribution to any significant training programme. Training, especially initial induction, was recognised as of considerable importance by the service. The basic grade staff were definitely *not* being employed as simple care or domestic assistants; their job description made it clear that they were to carry responsibility 'for providing personal care, training, education, recreation and friendship' to the residents in their house. Given that a proportion of the workforce would have little or no experience, an intensive induction course was a high priority. Our first survey was conducted before the appointment of the training officer so we anticipated some differences between staff who had received an induction and those, appointed a little later, who had not.

3 Patterns of Employment

This chapter is concerned not only with the kinds of people who were employed in the two organisations but also with the ways in which the different kinds of people fitted into those organisations. We shall describe the basic demographic characteristics of the staff and relate these to the patterns of working, before going on to examine the motivations and expectations that staff displayed. We shall also relate the motivations of staff to the recruitment process and the adaption of staff to working in their challenging new jobs.

Workforce composition

As we saw in the last chapter, one of the aims of the community service was to provide a reasonable mix of staff in terms of sex and age, given that the residents in the staffed houses were mixed. Something approaching equal proportions of men and women was the target, and, at the time of the postal survey, 42 per cent of the community care staff were male. The rate of leaving the community service was the same for men and women, although it was subsequently mostly women who applied for the posts that were advertised. Maintaining this proportion may be problematic therefore. Certainly experience elsewhere suggests that the bulk of the workforce in such services is female; for example 77 per cent of those working in the Nimrod Scheme are women (Evans et al. 1984). Furthermore it is predominantly 'young women without children' who are said to apply because the low wages are unlikely to attract 'sole wage-earners' (Mansell et al. 1987, p.110). However, the situation is almost certainly more complex than this and may depend to some extent on the ways in which given levels of earnings can be obtained. We shall return to this point later in this section.

The proportion of women working in the hospital also was high at 71 per cent but, as we shall relate, these were not mostly 'young women without children'. In the hospital men were in a minority and were not represented evenly in the different grades and shifts, or in terms of part-time working arrangements. In fact most male staff were qualified. The proportion of all *qualified* staff who were male was 42 per cent, while only a small number of men were unqualified nursing assistants. In this respect the community service had apparently matched the sex composition of the qualified part of the hospital workforce but had achieved this at a more basic care level. The working conditions of men and women in the community service were the same but the variety of possible working patterns in the hospital had led historically to very different sub-groups within that organisation. Table 3.1 gives the proportions of the care staff in the hospital who worked in groups defined by either the shift or the hours worked.

Table 3.1
Proportions of total hospital staff in each shift/time working group (per cent)

Day shift:	70.8	*Night shift:*	29.2
Comprising		Comprising	
Full time:	62.4	Full time:	11.9
Part time:	8.4	Part time:	17.3

The hospital needed half as many staff on duty at night as it did in the day. More than half of the night staff worked part time and the majority were women: 32.9 per cent of the day staff but only 18.6 per cent of the night staff were men. In our survey there were only two men among the part timers. Thus male staff in the hospital were typically qualified, full time employees working on the day shifts.

The age distributions in the two organisations were also noticeably different. Figure 3.1 presents these distributions for all the community staff compared with hospital care staff from charge nurse/sister to nursing assistant level. Because the latter comprise the bulk of the workforce, the age distribution for assistants alone would look virtually the same as that shown in the figure for all hospital care staff. There are two features of this comparison

Figure 3.1

Distribution of age groups in the two services

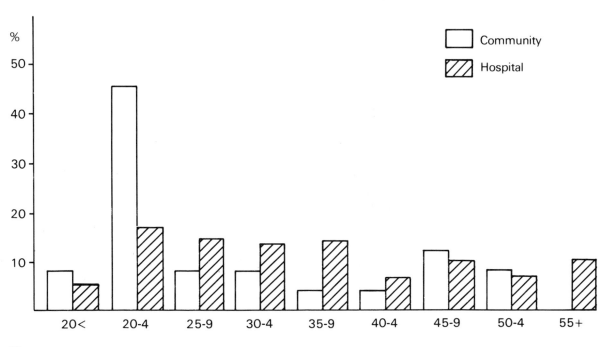

which are important. Firstly, we note the disproportionate contribution of young people to the community service. Nearly half of those who worked in staffed houses were in the 20–24 age band. This partially reflects what was said above about the typical work force in community schemes. Detailed comparison with the experience in the Nimrod service, for example, is difficult because they report wider age bands, but nearly half the staff employed in that scheme were under 29 (Evans, 1984). Thus there is a considerable difference in the average age of the two sets of staff: 35.9 years in the hospital, but only 29.9 years in the community service.

Secondly, Figure 3.1 shows that at the time of the study the community service, by comparison with the hospital, was not attracting employees in the middle age groups. Among the other age groups staff were represented in similar proportions in the hospital and in the Community. It was in the middle years, from 25 to 44, that the community was different. It might be argued that the community pattern reflected the difficulties faced by young women with children, were it not that women of this age group were well represented in the hospital. Within the community service there were no significant differences in the way men and women were distributed by age and no difference in the average age of the two sexes. This similarity within the community was presumably a product of the lack of differential working patterns, but in the hospital the working patterns of male and female staff in the middle age bands were quite different. This suggests that different working arrangements would be needed to fill the under-represented age groups in the community, if that was a desired aim.

Explaining the different employment patterns of men and women has most often relied on analysis of the implications of marriage and the presence of dependent children. For example, there are established effects in the case of the turnover of nurses (Mercer, 1979). Clearly, in the case of the community service it was people in the mid-life, child rearing part of the life-cycle who were under-represented. In fact, at the time of the survey, none of the community staff had any dependent children, while in the hospital over a third (36 per cent) of the staff reported at least one dependent child.

We have already shown that male hospital staff characteristically worked full time and further analysis confirmed that there were no significant effects due to age connected with the shift work pattern or the presence of dependent children. There was an effect on shift working, however, in that men on the night shift were twice as likely to have dependent children. For female staff the situation was rather different. With so many different factors involved it is difficult to make sense of the situation without some organising principle. Probably the most illuminating approach is to view the circumstances of groups of staff as the cause of the individual's strategic employment choices. This is the rationale for the form of Table 3.2 which shows the patterns of employment chosen by women with and without children. Just over a third (34.9 per cent) of all female staff had at least one dependent child, and this is the same as the proportion found amongst all categories of nurses nationally (NUPE, 1987).

Table 3.2

Average ages and proportions of women hospital care staff, with or without children, working in different shift/time patterns

	Shift (%)		Time worked	Per cent of staff with/ without children	Average age in (years)	Per cent of total staff
Staff with dependent children (100 per cent)	Day shifts	47	Full time	35	(31)	8
			Part time	12	(35)	3
	Night shift	53	Full time	16	(40)	4
			Part time	37	(35)	9
Staff without dependent children (100 per cent)	Day shifts	77	Full time	68	(29)	30
			Part time	8	(57)	4
	Night shift	23	Full time	8	(50)	4
			Part time	15	(49)	6

The final column in Table 3.2 gives the proportion of the total staff complement, including men, that each group represents. It is clear that, for example, young women without children working full time day shifts constitute the largest single category among women but comprise only 30 per cent of the total staff at the hospital. Women with at least one dependent child comprise nearly a quarter (24 per cent) of the total staff. Naturally women with dependent children fall within the middle age bands and, as the table shows, their average ages do not vary much across the possible categories of employment. The differences shown are probably due to chance. For women without dependent children, however, the choice of employment pattern is clearly age dependent. The difference centres on the choice of full time day work versus all other categories. We can most effectively summarize these findings by saying that once women with at least one dependent child have decided to work at the hospital their choice of work pattern is not directly affected by their age, but, if they have no dependent children then they tend to work full time day shifts if young and make some other arrangement if older.

The distribution of age groups of those without dependent children working full time is almost identical to the pattern reported for the community, so this is a clear indication that the possibilities at the hospital for various different patterns of working, permit the employment of women of different ages. It is mostly the choice of shift which separates these groups. Younger women without dependent children are less prepared to choose night work.

Women with children choose in roughly equal proportions whether to work day or night shifts, but show clear preferences for either full time day work or part-time night work. These choices are almost certainly based on a combination of economic and domestic factors. The average for part-time hours worked at night was 30.6 compared to 27.2 hours on part-time day shift but night work pay was significantly higher, so that part-time night work represents a good bargain for a woman with children. The average time quoted above is approximately equivalent to three nights. In our survey the average earnings of nursing assisants working part-time nights were 9.8 per cent *higher* than assistants on full time day shifts, so women working full time days could maintain their earnings, once their domestic circumstances included children, by changing to part-time night work. Clearly the level of earnings is important but it is the flexibility in employment opportunities that enables so many women to do some work in the hospital. There were four different patterns of part-time night shift hours in our survey and eleven different patterns of part-time day-shifts. Altogther, as Table 3.2 shows, over a fifth of the total staff complement were women who worked part-time.

The hospital is clearly an organisation which is largely staffed by women without dependent children but its organisational flexibility, in terms of available working patterns, has enabled it to retain women from all age groups, whereas, in the community service, such women have proved difficult to recruit. Male employees, on the other hand, are not apparently attracted by such part-time arrangements and recruiting them or at least retaining them, especially at basic grade, is probably not possible without a higher salary base. At this point, therefore, we have begun to raise the issue of career structure. We will return to the development of careers in Chapter Seven. Here we report on the backgrounds and experience of staff as these affect current and future employment.

Clearly professional qualifications are important in this employment market but, in both types of service, the care staff are mostly unqualified. In this circumstance it is probably relevant experience that structures the available labour pool. Table 3.3 sets out the kinds of qualifications reported by staff in both organisations.

Table 3.3
Professional qualifications of community and hospital staff (per cent)

	Community staff	Hospital staff
Registered nurse MH (includes RNMS)	12.5	30.0
Enrolled nurse	12.5	12.0
Social work qualification	17.0	0.5
Other	4.0	1.0
None	54.0	57.0

In addition to these qualifications, eight per cent of the community staff and 19 per cent of the hospital staff quoted a further qualification. In the community these were social work qualifications (CSS); in the hospital 5 per cent had other nursing qualifications (especially general), 3 per cent preliminary social care, 2 per cent nursery nursing and 11 per cent other. As Table 3.3 shows, there was only one major difference in the distribution of professional qualifications between the organisations. The community service employed about half as many registered nurses and made up the difference in qualified staff by employing people with a social work qualification. The proportions of unqualified staff were virtually identical.

What previous experience did the staff have? Were there differences within groups that reflected different aspects of the two services? In Table 3.4 we report the distribution of previous main occupations. These proportions represent answers to a question about the last main job before beginning work in the mental handicap field and excluded brief jobs or part-time work.

Table 3.4
Previous main job of qualified and unqualified staff in community and hospital (per cent)

	Community		Hospital	
	Qualified	Unqualified	Qualified	Unqualified
Present job is first job	9	15	21	26
Previous job with people with mental handicaps	73	15	19	6
Similar service occupation	—	8	14	17
Other sorts of work	18	62	46	51

Two points in Table 3.4 deserve attention. The first is that, in both organisations, the pattern of experience of qualified staff is, not surprisingly perhaps, different from that of unqualified staff ($p < .05$) in that the qualified staff are more likely to have spent all their working life working with this client group. However, between the organisations the experience of qualified staff is very different ($p < .001$). In the community very few qualified staff have experience outside the field, and this finding reflects the average age of this group. In the hospital, by contrast, nearly half the qualified staff report a previous main occupation in some field other than the care of mentally handicapped people. The pattern of previous experience amongst unqualified staff was not different between organisations, the differences in the table being chance fluctuations.

These findings are another reflection of the newness of the community service. Its qualified staff are mostly younger, with an average age of 25.7 years, compared with the unqualified staff at 33.5 years ($p < .05$). It is the unqualified staff in the community service who therefore have the wider occupational experience. In the hospital the qualified staff are not, on average, significantly different in age from their unqualified colleagues and similar proportions from each category have had experience at some time of other sorts of work. As Table 3.4 shows, most staff had had other jobs before their present one, the majority in entirely different sorts of occupation.

Of those with previous experience in working with people with mental handicaps, how many have already worked in a community setting? Amongst hospital staff, of course, very few (4 per cent) but in the community service, a quarter (25 per cent) had previously worked in some other community setting and half (50 per cent) had had previous experience in a hospital. Amongst present hospital staff 22 per cent had had experience of some other hospital.

For the latter group a degree of geographical mobility is obviously indicated. In the community the employment of local people, who know the area, is often part of the philosophy of the service, se we might expect less mobility in that service. In the interviews we asked the staff to describe their work histories and we included questions about geographical mobility. Within the community there was no difference between the qualified and unqualified staff: almost all the staff had been locally resident at the time they had taken the job. In Table 3.5, all the community staff are thus grouped together for comparison with qualified and unqualified hospital staff.

Table 3.5
Mobility of staff for present job (per cent)

	Community	Hospital	
	All staff	Qualified	Unqualified
Local	77	40	81
Moved within county	12	34	14
Moved from outside county	12	25	5

The pattern for the hospital is what would be expected for nurses, given their long established reputation for such mobility (Harris, 1963). The unqualified staff were drawn almost entirely from the local area and, given the average earnings and prevalence of part-time working, this is what would be expected. Within the community the qualified staff had largely been drawn from the hospital but had generally not moved to that job from outside the region. The community service was therefore a much more locally based service in this respect, but, of course, the great majority of hospital staff were unqualified and of local origin so, overall, the difference was not so great. Only 15 per cent of the total hospital sample had moved from outside the county to take their present job.

Motivations

Having a highly motivated staff would seem to be an obvious benefit to any service organisation, but there are clearly interactions between motivations, expectations and subsequent experience. Performance related motivation is discussed in later chapters where reactions to job and work roles are examined; here our concern is more with the sorts of motives which people brought to the service. For our present purposes the importance of motivation is the light that it may shed on job choice. Where there is a high and constant demand for staff, for example due to high turnover, the occupational choice of employees assumes relatively greater significance. We can approach motivation of this sort in several ways. We asked about first contact with the client group, about the reasons for working with mentally handicapped people, about how staff got their jobs and about motivation and identity with the career. We then asked people about their expectations and adaptations to the jobs

Different degrees of career orientation may be reflected in the mechanism of job choice. Hockey (1976 p. 125) compares 'vocational' nurses with those 'influenced' by others or by experience, and 'drifters' who have minimal reasons for entering the profession. Mercer (1979 pp. 136–8) classifies recruitment motivations somewhat differently, comparing orientations equivalent to the 'vocational' category with those revealing a basic instrumental approach. Other qualitatively different orientations within the vocational or professional category have been suggested for nurses (Matz, 1969) but, in the context of a major change in the nature and organisation of the work, rather different professional ideologies might be expected in the different organisations (c.f. Strauss et al. 1964). We report in detail on these latter aspects of the situation in the next chapter since the possibility of discordant beliefs may be one factor that motivates a proportion of the hospital staff to move to community service.

Regardless of more complex belief patterns, in terms of job choice we would expect differences between qualified and unqualified staff in both organisations, and, possibly, between organisations. Thus our intention in the interviews was to explore the reasons why these groups of staff had originally chosen to work with mentally handicapped people. Our classification of these motivations appears in Table 3.6.

Table 3.6

The reasons for working with people with mental handicap given by community staff, qualified and unqualified hospital staff (per cent)

	All community staff	Qualified hospital staff	Unqualified hospital staff
Extrinsic reasons	—	5	45
Career	29	58	5
Intrinsic reasons	41	11	41
Other	29	26	9

The distinction between extrinsic and intrinsic rewards was first introduced by Herzberg et al. (1959). Extrinsic features of work include money, security and so on, whilst intrinsic elements relate to such subjective aspects as opportunities for accomplishment. The notion of career as we have interpreted it here, includes aspects of both extrinsic and intrinsic motivations but is linked to the usual notion of progressive development. Accidental or other minimal motivations are collected in the final category. We do not assume in this analysis that the motivations underlying job choice necessarily have implications for job performance or organisational commitment (Daniel, 1969). Indeed a dramatic change in career is indicated by the move from hospital to community.

There are several ways in which these data could be presented but we have given them in this form to highlight the fact that the community staff, as a whole, are more like the qualified section of the hospital staff, in that both groups give priority to reasons other than extrinsic. Within the community, there are further comparisons which can be made. For example there were no real differences attributable to hospital experience. Career type motivation was present to the same degree amongst those with no hospital experience. There was a small difference ($p < .1$) between qualified and unqualified staff within the community, in that the unqualified staff tended not to speak in terms of a career, but instead highlighted the intrinsic elements of the occupation. For qualified staff in both organisations, the pattern was much the same, and indeed was similar to that found in the nursing profession in general (Hockey, 1976, p 125).

The major differences then, are between the hospital nursing assistants and all other staff. For assistants the job choice was overall more deliberate, in that very few mentioned accidental factors leading to their taking up the work. The more or less equal proportions giving either extrinsic or intrinsic reasons reflected two basic job choice strategies. For some the possibility of shift-work or part-time work, or simply any work, was the main attraction. For others the extra interest or challenge of a job which paid much the same as a range of semi-skilled occupations, had been the deciding factor. Unqualified staff employed in the community fell mostly into this latter category. Consonant with the aim of setting up a new and innovatory form of care the community service had clearly recruited people on the basis of their motivation to do intrinsically more interesting work. Amongst our interviewees, this meant at least a long term commitment to care work and, usually, a commitment to the client group.

What were the origins of this commitment? With a fairly high and constant demand for basic staff it is useful to know what mechanisms had first brought this form of work to the attention of the staff. When the answers to questions about first contact with mentally handicapped people were classified another parallel between community staff and the qualified section of the hospital staff emerged. The largest single source of contact for all staff was with the present job but, whilst qualified staff reported this the least (22 per cent), and community staff slightly more (35 per cent), half the nursing assistants gave this response. For qualified hospital staff and community staff, the origins of motivation generally predated the current job. These results were consistent with the job choice analysis and underline the importance of some prior contact with the client group. Indeed the nature of first contact, for example, informal vs. institutional, may well be the basis for differences in the subsequent beliefs staff have about people with mental handicap (St Claire, 1986). It has been found that people with a mentally handicapped relative for example, may subsequently be motivated to work in the field (Carr, 1985). Table 3.7 sets out the various mechanisms of first contact in order of degree of effect.

Table 3.7
First contact with mentally handicapped people (per cent all interviewees)

Present job only	36.8
Experience in own community, school, etc.	21.1
Told by relatives or friends	17.5
On placement from a course	10.5
Whilst doing other (unrelated) type of work	7.0
By family experience	7.0

Recruitment

The process of recruitment too, varied between, on the one hand, unqualified staff in the hospital and, on the other hand, qualified staff in the hospital and all the community staff. Recent research has shown that finding a job is often mediated by some informal contact with or knowledge of, the employing organisation (MSC, 1984). In this study quite active informal recruitment was described by many of our hospital interviewees, especially those who were unqualified. It was not just that knowledge of the hospital, or more usually of someone already employed there, contributed to the choice of work. Quite often people described their recruitment to the type of work as a process involving persuasion. The following is perhaps the most extreme example, but similar stories were not uncommon.

'A friend of mine started work here on the night shift and a while later she suggested that I might try it. But I was not at all for the idea—I was frightened of it. It took her about three months to persuade me until I started work here just for the two nights. I liked it then.'

(Long service nursing assistant)

In contrast the community staff and the qualified hospital staff tended to be self motivated, as Table 3.8 suggests.

Table 3.8
Nature of job recruitment (per cent)

	All community staff	Qualified hospital staff	Unqualified hospital staff
Applied blind without other contact	71	53	14
Contact with organisation in another capacity (eg different job on site)	—	11	—
Via informal contact with third party	29	37	86

Clearly earlier contact with people with mental handicaps, reported by community and qualified staff, helped to motivate them to work with this client group. Although the increasing numbers of people with mental handicaps being cared for in the community may increase the likelihood of contact little can actually be done to enhance such a chance effect, which suggests that advertising of posts should be as wide as possible. However, there are two other possible interventions which could improve the supply of staff. One is to recognise the contribution made by those college courses which arrange for visits and placements across a range of client groups. The value of any course which provides direct contact with a client group to young people who may not have a firm occupational direction is evident from the responses shown in the above three tables. The Preliminary Certificate in Social Care (PCSC), which was recognised by the local authority covered by our research, was mentioned by those staff who possessed it as the origin of their interest. Thus the labour supply function of placement is of considerable value and the PCSC would seem to be a particularly valuable example of this.

The second possible avenue is to recognise the contribution of informal networks amongst employees. The hospital, given its large size and multiplicity of different occupations, tended to be seen as a local industry by many of its unqualified staff. This does not mean, however, that the quality of their motivation was automatically to be devalued. As we reported above (Table 3.6), the proportion who claimed to have chosen the work because of its nature was almost the same as the proportion who mentioned only extrinsic rewards. Again the problem is one of experience. For hospital staff the likelihood of knowing somebody who already had experience of the job was quite high. The local nature of the labour pool enhanced this effect.

Even in the community, the informal contacts shown on Table 3.8 had often been made through the hospital, in that ex-hospital employees had helped recruit one another to the new type of service. Obviously this process cannot survive the closure of the hospital, but, during the closure period, it is probable that a proportion of the staff would want to move into community employment. For qualified staff this decision will be coloured by career considerations and professional ideology. As we reported, the 'career' orientation of qualified staff was not under-represented in the community compared to the hospital, so belief in the viability of a career in the local authority structure was firm. For unqualified staff, a move to the community might be encouraged by contact with people already employed in such a service, as was the case for some of our interviewees. Their motivation tended to be different from that of their qualified colleagues, but, as we showed above, need not be assumed to be merely extrinsic.

The proportion of unqualified staff in the hospital with an entirely 'self-propelled' orientation to work is quite small, so that methods of augmenting informal contact might be successful in attracting staff with hospital experience. Korman and Glennerster (1984 pp. 146–7) discuss the possibility of secondment of staff from new (or planned) facilities back to the parent hospital so that transition of staff and residents might be better conducted. However, they noted the reluctance of staff to move, and attributed this to uncertainty about the hospital's future. More probably such reluctance is a characteristic of labour forces generally, especially in the case of a well established organisation providing a variety of occupational opportunities to a local area. In other words, the inertia of the staff was a function of its composition, which was largely unqualified with a considerable number of part-time and relatively immobile women. Unqualified staff living near to a community development would probably benefit by savings on transport, for example, but unless the community service could offer a variety of employment options many female staff would be unwilling or unable to make the transition. This would be true even if they were made aware of the nature of the work by, for example, a joint community/hospital initiative arranged at villa level in the hospital.

We were interested in knowing what had motivated staff to take up work which involved caring for people with mental handicaps. As one nursing assistant said 'I wanted to do something worthwhile and not just fiddle with bits of paper'. We attempted to estimate the degree of involvement which the staff felt: Table 3.9 gives the results. It shows that the main differences were again between qualified and unqualified staff. The differences between the hospital and the community, which we found in other parts of the analysis, did not show up here. For the majority of the qualified staff their work was a major aspect of their lives, while a majority of the unqualified staff had only a partial or marginal involvement in their jobs.

Table 3.9
Involvement of staff in caring work as an aspect of their lives (per cent of interview responses)

	All qualified staff	All unqualified staff
A major aspect of life	61	38
Career orientation	18	7
Partial or marginal involvement	21	55

(The differences are not due to chance: $p < .05$)

The differences shown here are hardly surprising, given the investment that qualified staff make in their careers. However, the view of work that people have when they enter it need not have implications for their subsequent behaviour, in terms for example, of whether they stay or leave. As we reported in Chapter Two, the community service actually had a higher rate of turnover than the hospital. So that despite the evidence of high motivation retention was a major problem. There were no differences in rates of turnover between qualified and unqualified staff. We will discuss the factors which contribute to turnover in some detail in Chapter Seven. At this point, however, our discussion moves on to cover expectations. Clearly the nature of job choice and job performance are likely to interact with expectations. A member of staff from the community project said,

> 'I knew about mentally handicapped people from college (placement). I just saw an advert in the paper for the hospital and applied. On the day shift ... all the staff did was clear up and so on ... really boring things (Community service?) I knew (staff) and she told me about it. (Expectations?) I didn't know what to expect at the hospital, it was better than I thought it might be. (Community?) It was obviously going to be better ... I was told you'll be able to do all these wonderful things ... (Motivation?) Not in the hospital, too frustrating, you couldn't do what you wanted. (Community?). Too involved really ... there's no let up from it.'

This interviewee had followed through a motivation which had its origins in a college placement. She was not a qualified nurse and was reacting to her community job in an entirely different way from her experience in the hospital. Not surprisingly frustration in one setting was fuel for an enhanced expectation of the new service but, in fact, this respondent was still struggling with her actual experience and had not fully adapted to the community role.

Expectations and Adaptations

What sort of knowledge did staff have of the conditions of the work? We have shown that many people were recruited by informal contact and that qualified staff especially had often had more direct early experience of the client group, so we might expect their foreknowledge to be greater. Certainly appointment to the community service was more likely for people with some experience of working with mentally handicapped people, and as Table 3.4 showed, the majority of the community staff had had experience of this kind. When we classified the responses to questions about expectations several sorts of differences appeared.

Firstly, there were no real differences within the community; yet again there was a certain homogeneity in that service. In the hospital, however, there was a difference between qualified and unqualified staff. As can be seen in Table 3.10, this difference concerned surprise or shock reactions to the conditions.

Table 3.10
Nature of expectations concerning the job (per cent of interview responses)

	All community staff	Qualified hospital staff	Unqualified hospital staff
More or less accurate	18	6	9
Some knowledge	65	35	36
Very unsure	—	6	41
Shock and/or surprise	18	53	14

(The differences are not due to chance: $p < .01$)

The experience of the community staff on the one hand, and the informal recruitment of unqualified hospital staff on the other, meant that prior knowledge of the likely conditions was quite high. Thus we could assume that adaptation to the community job would be facilitated by this knowledge and experience, and the informally communicated knowledge of many assistants would also enable them to adapt. This was the pattern that further staff responses confirmed at interview. Table 3.11 sets these responses out for the same groups.

Table 3.11
Adaptation to the present job (per cent of interview responses)

	All community staff	Qualified hospital staff	Unqualified hospital staff
Well prepared	53	12	9
Adapted quickly	—	53	46
Adapted slowly	35	29	46
Currently struggling	12	6	—

(The differences are not due to chance: $p < .001$)

In addition to these results it was not surprising to discover that the ex-hospital staff within the community generally thought themselves well prepared. As Table 3.10 showed, however, there were few community staff whose expectations were accurate, so there was considerable scope for dissatisfaction. These interviewees were all 'survivors' of course, so that, whether they had adapted quickly or slowly, all had remained in the organisation at least long enough to be interviewed. Stories abounded in the hospital of staff who left on the first day, or after a few days, and although these were probably exaggerated organisational myths, the experience of the community service did include one or two people who had simply left without any formal explanation. We might speculate that the many staff who had some informal prior contact with the job were encouraged by such connections to remain long enough to adapt to it. Realistic information of this sort can reduce the tendency to quit early (Wanous, 1980). In the hospital there was a common belief that if you stayed a week you could stay as long as you liked, which suggests a fairly sharp form of the 'induction crisis' that has been argued to be a feature of most employment (see Bryant, 1965). As we suggested above, and illustrated with a quotation from a long service part-time assistant and with the data of Table 3.8, unqualified entrants to the hospital typically had informal medi- ation through this process. For those without such support some form of induction training is probably the only effective organisational intervention that can assist in this adaptation to work.

The results shown in Table 3.11 also emphasise that the community job could present a considerable challenge to staff. Just under half of our community interviewees had experienced, or were experiencing, problems in coming to terms with the work. Nor was this division exclusively centred on those with or without previous experience. The demands of the job are different. Thus even an ex-hospital nurse, who claimed to be well prepared for the *better environment* of the community, was surprised by the demands made on staff.

4 Ideology and Suitability

In this chapter we turn our attention to beliefs about the nature of the work and the 'appropriate' forms of service. Whatever staff expectations might be, in order to do the job, or to continue doing the job, people's motivation and beliefs need to be in some sort of equilibrium. Given that the kinds of motivation we have recorded in the previous chapter were rather varied we might expect, for example, that self-selection from hospital into community jobs would occur amongst people who approved in one way or another the ideas associated with that form of service.

There are two sets of attitudes which are relevant in this context. Firstly, there are attitudes towards people with mental handicap themselves, especially in terms of their supposed abilities and potential, and, secondly, there are attitudes towards alternative models of care. There has been an assumption in some previous research, exemplified by Jones (1975), that lack of belief in the potential of people with mental handicap is related to reduced levels of performance in teaching and social aspects of care by care staff. There is some evidence of a relationship between staff attitudes, and care practices (Pratt et al, 1980). It was not our intention to pursue this kind of inquiry; however, it seemed likely that beliefs about mentally handicapped people and about appropriate care would influence the decisions members of staff made about their own employment. To anticipate our discussion, in Chapter Seven, concerning factors affecting the likelihood of staff turnover and orientations towards taking-up community work, we note that staff are differentially mobile in occupational and geographical terms. Thus the presence of a strong belief in favour of community care amongst, for example, younger members of staff, could have considerable significance for their subsequent tendency to leave, whilst such a belief amongst more senior staff might instead be very important in facilitating co-operation between services.

Orientations and Beliefs

The survey commissioned by the Jay Committee (Jay Report, Vol. 2, 1979) adopted the approach developed by Jones (1975) and produced a new version of her scale of 'Treatment Orientation'. This scale was designed to provide a score for staff which represented their degree of 'optimism' about the potential of people with mental handicap to learn and develop. The purposes of the Jay survey were to compare the staff's views with 'those implicit in the Government's white paper'. The Jay survey found more 'optimism' than Jones, whose data had been collected in 1972, but it could not conclude that there had been a real change because the scales used were not strictly comparable. Given the fairly dramatic developments in the provision of care that have subsequently occurred, our postal questionnaire included a similar scale. The Jay survey also developed a scale to measure the value attached to community care. It found that community (hostel) staff were more favourable towards the provision of community care, as were the more senior staff within hospitals. No relationship was found between the levels of ability of residents and staff orientation towards community care provision. The survey also established a correlation between these scales in that staff who were more 'optimistic' about the abilities of people with mental handicap also tended to believe in the appropriateness of community care.

We drew items from these sources and developed two scales which we called Resident Orientation and Service Orientation. In addition we added three separate questions on the likelihood of certain outcomes of policy. Our assumption in developing measures of this sort was that attitudes towards either resident characteristics or service options would each fall on one major dimension. This is the basic assumption underpinning all such scales, where each separate item is treated as essentially a slightly different measure of the same underlying thing (Ghiselli et al, 1984). We shall re-examine these assumptions later in this section. In addition to community staff our analysis distinguished between nursing assistants (NA), state enrolled nurses (EN) state registered nurses (RN), charge nurses/sisters (CN/S) and nursing officers (NO).

In general our findings confirmed those reported by the Jay survey. There was an overall tendency for positive agrreement between the scales, in that staff who had a more progressive attitude towards the residents also supported the development of community services. However, this effect was *absent* amongst community staff, enrolled nurses and charge nurse/ sisters. It was not surprising to discover, as we report below, that community staff scored very much higher than hospital staff on both these scales, but the lack of a significant relationship between the scales amongst these staff is equivalent to saying that their judgement of resident potential had no implications for their judgement of service options.

Figure 4.1 displays the scores on the two scales for the community staff as a whole and for the different grades of hospital staff. The vertical line represents the overall average score of all groups and bars to the right indicate (a) more progressive attitudes towards residents; (b) stronger support for community based services. Three differences are of importance. Firstly, the community staff scored higher than the hospital staff on both scales. Secondly, however, the community staff score on the Resident Orientation scale was not sufficiently different from three groups within the hospital, namely staff nurses, sisters and senior nurses, for the difference to be attributable to anything other than chance. In the case of Service Orientation, the score of the community staff was similar to the score achieved by senior nurses. Thirdly, as was reported by the Jay survey and others (Moores and Grant, 1976), nursing assistants and state enrolled

Figure 4.1

Resident and service orientations of community staff and of different grades of hospital staff

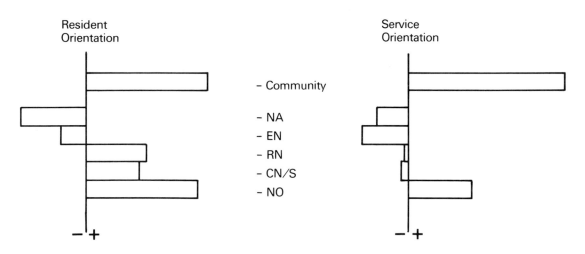

Bars to the right of the vertical lines indicate:
a) more progressive attitudes towards residents (see Question 33 in the Appendix)
b) stronger support for community services (see Question 36 in the Appendix)

nurses had the most 'pessimistic' view of residents and it was these same groups who were least in favour of the community service. In fact, as the figure shows, there was a pronounced trend within the hospital for Resident Orientation to become more progressive with increasing seniority (p<.001), and there was a similar, though less striking trend in the case of Service Orientation (p<.05).

Within the community we examined the responses on these two scales for variations between qualified and unqualified staff and between groups defined by their previous hospital experience, or lack of it. In the first comparison, by qualifications, there were no differences on either scale. When we compared staff with and without hospital experience, however, regardless of their former grade, there were differences. Exactly half the community staff had had experience of hospital work and this group had a *more* progressive view of residents than their colleagues who had had no experience, or had had experience only of other community work (p<.05). Similarly those with hospital experience were slightly more in favour of the community service idea, although statistically the difference in this case could well have been due to chance (p<.1).

Following the logic of the Resident Orientation scale as originally envisaged, that is to say as a scale which measures variation due to experience with residents of differing ability (Jones, 1975), we analysed both scales to see if either or both were related to resident characteristics. In the hospital neither the level of perceived dependency nor the proportion of residents with behaviour problems on the villa or unit had any relationship with the scores for Resident or Service Orientation. Views on these things were held independently of the level of dependency or the proportion of behaviour problems. This is not too surprising, of course, since many staff would have had experience in more than one setting within the hospital as a whole. In the community, however, there was an effect on Service Orientation. Whereas the generally progressive view of residents remained unaffected by the resident characteristics, belief in the appropriateness of care in a community service was less when there were more residents with behaviour problems.

Was there a parallel to this in beliefs about what would happen to mental handicap services in the future? The three further questions we included were intended to tap views about the likelihood of certain outcomes, rather than their appropriateness or desirability. Community and hospital staff disagreed about the chances of two out of three outcomes, as shown in Table 4.1.

Table 4.1
Likelihood of various policy outcomes (average scores)

Outcome (scored 1 for very unlikely 5 for very likely)	Community	Hospital	Sig
1. That not all mentally handicapped people will be discharged into the community	3.8	3.6	n.s.
2. That the 'move to the community' will produce a poor service	2.1	3.4	$p < .0001$
3. That the public will accept mentally handicapped people in the community	3.6	2.4	$p < .0001$

Not surprisingly the community staff were optimistic about their own kind of service surviving to produce a valuable form of care, and they believed, on the basis of some experience, of course, that the public would accept their clients. Hospital staff were less convinced that these things would happen, even though their own institution was subject to an advanced closure plan and had already shut down villas. Both groups agreed, however, in their response to statement number one; neither group of staff thinks it very likely that *all* residents will be discharged. So, to return to the question, how did beliefs about appropriate services relate to estimates of likely outcomes? Within the hospital, statements two and three were related to Service Orientation, in that those who believed in the appropriateness of community care also thought it unlikely that that kind of service would produce poor results and were optimistic about public response. Amongst community staff, however, estimates of the likelihood of these outcomes were not related to views about the appropriateness of community care. Just as views about the potential of people with mental handicap were independent of views on appropriate types of service, so too were estimates of outcomes.

Statement one, concerning the discharge of all residents, was not related to Service Orientation either for community or hospital staff. Furthermore, whilst all groups judged statements two and three consistently, seeing both as more or less likely, no group judged the likelihood of statement number one as in any way related to the other outcomes. As Table 4.1 suggests, there was a widespread belief that a proportion of residents would remain in some form of hospital care, and this view did not vary in relation to other beliefs. We can summarize these findings by saying that, within the hospital, there was varying commitment to community care but a widespread belief that it would probably not take over completely, whilst in the community there was a very strong and uniform belief in community care, but similar doubts about it eventually serving all the potential residents.

As we explained above, in the first phase of the research we followed the logic of previous inquiries, such as the Jay survey, and conceived of a single dimension of views concerning community care; crudely we thought staff might be for it or against it. Clearly, however, these results suggest rather more complexity in staff views. To test our assumptions, we examined the pattern of responses to the two sets of eight items which made up the orientation scales to see if staff were judging the items in a related way. We used principal components analysis for this task. The technique examines each item's relationship with every other item. If our assumptions are correct, all the items should be related in the same sort of way, so that for example, agreement with Item 1 is usually paired with agreement or disagreement on Item 2 and so on. This was the case for Resident Orientation and we concluded that residents were seen by staff as having more or less potential on a single sliding scale. The scale for Service Orientation, however, divided into two separate parts; one linked statements which were pro-hospital or anti-community and one linked all the pro-community statements. In other words, staff tended to respond to the two forms of service in parallel, rather than as alternatives, and this, of course, is consistent with the widespread view that a proportion of the resident population will never be discharged.

When we discussed the forms of care in the interviews, we encountered a wide variety of comments. This section of the discussion was usually the longest and staff used the opportunity to express their concern and their, frequently complex, views about policies and their implementation. One of the ways in which we ordered this discussion was to ask staff what they thought should happen. Amongst community staff there were really only two kinds of responses to these questions. Staff either completely agreed with a full community service, provided for all available clients, or thought that a tiny proportion should be cared for in some specialist form of unit. The tiny proportion was defined by reference to violence and severe behaviour problems. Here are two quotations which represent these types of views. The first repudiates the isolation of problems.

[Is what you've said true of all hospital residents?]

'Yes, they should all come out. Property should be adapted. The only problems are violent people but there are plenty of such people in the community who aren't mentally handicapped.'

(Ex-enrolled nurse)

[What about all the residents in the hospital?]

'There are some I can't imagine ever moving out ... all I can imagine them moving to is like a hostel with lots of staff, run similar to a hospital, because they'll never ever change, they're so bad and violent too.'

(Ex-nursing assistant)

The public acceptability of certain residents is part of the rationale behind some of these replies but, in the hospital, the proportion of residents who were not thought suitable for community care was judged to be greater. However, it was not public acceptability so much as resident ability that underlay many of these replies.

[What about the policies behind the closure?]

'It's a good idea. Some of the people that are here should never have been here in the first place – but some of them, they don't know what they're going to. Some of the girls ... are quite intelligent and they could wander around the hospital but they wouldn't be able to do that in town – they haven't got the road sense and they probably never will have ...'

(Sister)

The most frequent response in the hospital was the 'some in, some out' approach, based on ability. In Table 4.2 we have summarized these sorts of belief patterns for the community and hospital staff separately. There were no real structural differences within the organisations, so that the various approaches within the hospital were distributed throughout the grades and by qualifications, while in the community there was little variation at all. The categories reflect what is illustrated above with the addition of two rather more 'institutional' types of response. Some hospital staff, whilst accepting that a few residents could leave, nevertheless felt that the rest should be accommodated in 'smaller units' within a hospital setting, and a few staff thought that the hospital should simply be improved. Underlying both these replies were arguments about the safety and dignity of residents: 'They are not ridiculed here'.

Table 4.2
Pattern of views on appropriate form of care (per cent of interview responses)

	Community staff	Hospital staff
Full community based system	47	2
Community system with minor special provision	41	17
'Some in, some out'	6	46
Smaller units within institutions	—	17
Other forms of improved institution	—	15
Don't know	6	2

We think it would be fair to characterise the principal difference between community and hospital staff's views as being based on two different kinds of judgement. Although, as Table 4.2 shows, a number of community staff doubted the possibility of a complete community service, the majority believed that all present residents should be discharged, regardless of their ability, as a matter of right. In the hospital, it was usually ability or potential that was the rationale for a belief in a partial community solution.

There are several important aspects to these findings. The first is that for most community staff the issue centred on the *rights* of people with mental handicap conceived in the manner of the first principle of the Jay Committee. Even so less than half the community staff were prepared to extend that principle to *all* possible clients. Beliefs of this sort, of course, specifically repudiate arguments about suitability and thus we have an explanation for the fact that the scores of community staff on the Resident Orientation scale were not strongly related to their scores on the Service Orientation scale.

Similarly, in the hospital, we can see that the overall relationship we reported between beliefs about resident potential and service provision reflects the 'some in, some out' philosophy that is the most likely response of the staff. Because, for hospital staff, the issue is largely one of *potential and ability* they see the provision of two sorts of service as a logical outcome, and this explains the partial decomposition of our Service Orientation scale into two parallel parts. Despite this difference, or perhaps because of it, there is one further important message in these findings. The majority of the hospital staff, at all levels, favoured at least some form of community service, as the first three categories of Table 4.2, totalling 65 per cent, clearly show.

Perhaps the greatest significance of this pattern of results is the potential for misunderstanding that it reveals. Whenever and wherever staff from the two kinds of organisation meet, to collaborate and co-ordinate the discharge of residents, or even informally, *the community staff will tend to conceive of the discharge of residents in terms of necessity, and hospital staff in terms of practicality.* Perhaps both sides need to know that (a) most hospital staff support the move to community care at least for a large proportion of residents and (b) most community staff expect special provision for some 'problem' residents.

Linked to the staffs' understandings of the forms of care are their views on their own role. We asked staff whether they saw their work role as most similar to the role of 'nurse', 'teacher' or 'carer'. Their answers displayed even more diversity than when we had asked about the future shape of the services. People whose careers could be greatly affected by their professional status displayed a considerable ambivalence about the 'nursing' aspect of the work. The qualified hospital staff were divided on the appropriateness of the label 'nurse' to define their role or their work. Less than half (44 per cent) adopted the label 'nurse' alone, while about the same number (38 per cent) avoided that term. The rest described their job as a mixed role. Only a minority (12 per cent) used the term 'carer', which was, by contrast, the term most often used by nursing assistants (46 per cent).

Whilst such terms tend to convey staffs' interpretations of the appropriate model of care, so that a majority of qualified staff do not see the job as much like 'normal nursing' or simple 'caring' but in more complex terms, their views on employment understandably emphasize their own suitability. The fear expressed by some was that in the community there was a prevalence of 'anti-nurse' feeling.

> 'I've had it said to me that it'll not be many people from the big hospitals that get the jobs in the community.'
>
> (Sister)

The irony is that the woman who made this remark could hardly be described as non-progressive. With very long service, and of an age to see out the closure programme to retirement, she nevertheless expressed views which favoured community care:

> [Residents] 'I could never understand why they were in hospital to start with'
>
> [Work Role] 'I couldn't understand why we were called nurses – it's a different kind of caring, training.'
>
> [Closure] 'There is some feeling of 'what's it all been for', because I think it's something that we never expected to happen. It is right that it is happening, as long as they look after the ones that are more handicapped.'

As this quotation, and the findings we have discussed suggest, there is a reservoir of feeling within the hospital which favours the current developments, but there is also concern that somehow the criticism of large institutions, which is implicit in current policies, has rubbed off onto the staff. The notion that care staff become 'institutionalised', in a parallel way to the process affecting residents (Raynes et al. 1979, p.117–120) may well have validity. For example our measure of Resident Orientation was negatively related to length of service so that longer service staff tended to see less potential in residents. But beliefs about the service options were *not* subject to this effect. Furthermore it is mostly younger staff who have the actual potential for movement between services and they are the least affected by the process. Finally, we are aware that there is a certain absurdity in the idea that whilst residents can be discharged from an institution and de-institutionalised for life in the community, their former professional caretakers may be seen as unsuitable employees because they are 'too institutionalised'. This point raises the issue of selection criteria for community employment.

Selection criteria and employment preferences

Several issues can be raised under this heading but the 'suitability' of hospital employees for community work is perhaps the most pressing. There are two major aspects to this topic: the nature of the skills possessed by staff and the willingness and/or availability of staff for community employment. To continue the theme of this chapter, which is concerned with the outlook of people employed in the two settings, we will address the latter aspects here and return to the nature of skills in Chapter Eight.

We have already recorded a considerable list of differences between community and hospital staff. Community staff were unlikely to be in the middle part of the life cycle, did not have dependent children and were mostly of local origin. Their basic motivations were like those of qualified staff in the hospital and, although the proportion with qualifications was the same, they were all very self-motivated people. Half of them had hospital experience but the overall pattern of their beliefs was similar to that of senior grade staff within the hospital. They were optimistic about public response and committed to community care for the large majority of residents. Clearly many of these characteristics have implications for the recruitment of staff; we noted that women with children for example, tended to prefer night shifts and part-time working. However, within such categories, defined by various practical considerations on the part of staff, there still remains the question 'Are staff likely to think of taking up community employment? As the quotation at the end of the previous section suggests, some staff fear that their suitability is partly judged on the basis of their supposed orientation towards the work. At the beginning of a service run-down, it might seem unlikely that staff with an institutional orientation would particularly *want* to seek community employment.

What did we learn about preferences and selection from our survey of staff in the two organisations? There are several related questions. What sort of hospital staff were employed in the community service? Who was selected? How many hospital staff match those who have transferred to the community? Are they likely to leave the hospital? What are the implications for the hospital if they do leave?

Obviously the community staff had *been* selected so the logically prior question is: to what extent were they self-selected? We asked the community service management specifically about the recruitment of hospital staff, and were told that none of the hospital applicants for whom we had data had failed to get a post if they had applied for one, although we learnt subsequently that some ex-hospital applicants had been rejected. Thus our group of ex-hospital community staff was essentially a self-selected group, and this permits us to ask the subsidiary questions.

The first of these concerns the proportion of hospital staff who might, at least in the initial stages, be candidates for the community service. We recognise that other community services could attract different sorts of people but we must limit our analysis to the staffed housing service. We reasoned that if the group of ex-hospital community staff was a self-selected group, then we could estimate the proportion of likely candidates amongst hospital staff by matching their characteristics to those of the self-selected group. We have already discussed the major differences of beliefs between the two organisations, but obviously within the hospital many people will have views more or less like the averages that we have compared and we wished to sort people by the pattern of their beliefs. We therefore combined several of our measures of beliefs using a technique called discriminant analysis.

Essentially this technique sorts out our measures according to which is the more effective in telling two groups apart. Then, using the values scored by community staff on those measures we traced the hospital staff who had the same pattern of responses.

The strongest differences were, first, on the Service Orientation scale, secondly, on the statement concerning the likelihood of the community giving a poor service, thirdly on the statement concerning public response and fourthly on the Resident Orientation scale. Taken together, this pattern of responses was matched by 22 per cent of the hospital staff. In other words, about a fifth of the staff in the hospital were so like the existing community staff that our measures could not tell them apart. Who were these people? We have already noted that Service Orientation and Resident Orientation changed systematically with seniority in the hospital. Thus the proportion of senior staff who matched the outlook of existing community staff was likely to be higher, and this was in fact the case.

Were they likely to take up community employment? We have two measures which are relevant to this question: Community Employment Orientation and Propensity to Leave. We discuss these measures more generally in Chapter Seven but, basically, the first measures the degree of likelihood of, and concern with, community employment and the second measures the likelihood and contemplation of leaving. We shall refer to the matched group of hospital staff as 'community-like'. When compared to the rest of the hospital staff this group did have a higher Propensity to Leave $(p<.05)$ and a marginally greater orientation towards community employment $(p<.1)$.

Thus it seems that staff who are in favour of the community type service, who see more potential in residents and believe the initiative is likely to succeed, are more ready to quit the hospital and, possibly, take up community employment. However, the presence of such views in greater proportion amongst senior grades argues against this, since, as we showed in Chapter Two, the leaving rate was fairly uniform throughout the hospital hierarchy. In other words, the higher average Propensity to Leave found in the community-like group is the result of a section of that group having a very high Propensity to Leave.

We do not need to speculate on the relative proportions involved, however, since we were able to check back, after an elapsed period of eighteen months, on who had subsequently left the hospital. Thus we can compare the proportions of staff in the 'community like' group with other hospital staff, and we can seek to confirm that the tendency to leave, as measured by the Propensity to Leave scale, did differ between sections of the 'community-like' group. Apart from the significance to community employers, who might wish to recruit from this group, the importance of this analysis is the light it sheds on the implications for the hospital during the closure programme. Table 4.3 sets out the proportions of the two sets of hospital staff in terms of who had left by the end of the study period.

Table 4.3
Proportions of 'stayers' and 'leavers' amongst 'community-like' hospital staff and others (per cent)

	Community-like hospital staff	All other hospital care staff
'Stayers'	64	83
'Leavers'	36	17

(The differences are not due to chance: p<.01)

The difference shown between the two types was considerable and was unlikely to be a chance effect. Over a third of the 'community-like' staff left at some time during the 18 month period. We could not obtain detailed information for the whole period on the destinations of these leavers but we can compare their scores on our scale of Orientation towards Community Employment. Amongst those who left, whom we have classified as 'community-like', the Orientation towards Community Employment was stronger than for those who left but were not particularly 'community-like' (p<.08). Note, however, that the latter were in the majority; nearly two-thirds of the leavers (62 per cent) were not 'community-like' staff.

To confirm our suggestion that 'community-like' staff might be best thought of as comprising two groups, those who were likely to leave and those were likely to stay, we compared the 'stayers' and 'leavers' within the 'community-like' type. The stayers were older, with an average age of 38.5 years compared to the leavers, whose average age was 31.6 years (p<.05). The 'stayers' also scored very much lower on the Propensity to Leave scale (5.8 compared with 7.4 for leavers; p<.05). Thus the 'community-like' staff comprised two groups: older, generally more senior people who were much less likely to leave, and younger mobile people who were very much more likely to leave, and possibly take up community employment.

The logic of this analysis is not startling but it does put some scale to the processes which are in train. One important implication concerns the composition of the work force over the period of closure. As Table 4.3 showed, there was a differential leaving rate for staff in the two groups. Figure 4.2 shows what this implied for the hospital as a whole over time.

As we saw in Chapter Two, the proportion of more dependent residents in the hospital increased in the first part of the closure programme, in line with the concerns expressed by Jones (1975 p.96). Here we see evidence of the parallel process that some practitioners have suggested, namely the gradual concentration of those more institutionally minded staff. However, these figures only describe leaving, not recruiting. Clearly new staff are being recruited, but as we noted in Chapter Two, fewer of the newly qualified staff are opting for hospital employment. There is almost certainly, then, a net loss of 'community-like' staff. How far will this process

Figure 4.2
Changes in the composition of the hospital workforce in terms of the proportion with different belief patterns over a period of 18 months

Time One

A	B
'Community-like' belief pattern 22 per cent	'Hospital' belief pattern 78 per cent

Losses

A	B
36 per cent	17 per cent

Time Two

A	B
'Community-like' belief pattern 18 per cent	'Hospital' belief pattern 83 per cent

go? If we simply assume an unchanging rate of leaving, then all such staff will have left before closure. But, as we have shown, most of the community-like staff are not especially likely to leave. Amongst 'stayers', in other words, there were no differences between the two types in terms of age, Propensity to Leave or Orientation towards Community Employment. The senior staff, who are disproportionately community minded, will increasingly lack like-minded young colleagues as the process of closure continues.

The corollary to this argument is that the total pool of hospital staff who are community-minded *and* likely to be available for community employment is probably quite small. The number of such people who left the hospital was only one-and-a-half times the total number who left the much smaller community service in the same period. As we indicated, it is not our intention to suggest that other staff, not presently sharing the same views as those we have labelled community-like, are somehow inappropriate employees. Rather it seems likely that those staff themselves will tend not to *choose* community employment. In fact the hospital provides an important route into mental handicap care work for the local labour pool. Recall that most unqualified staff were local and first worked with people with mental handicap at the hospital after entirely different forms of work, and that they relied heavily on informal contact with already employed staff in getting the work. A proportion of such people, actually 38 per cent, were what we have labelled community-like staff and 42 per cent of *them* had left during the period. In this sense, assuming that community employment was the destination of most of this, albeit small proportion, the hospital provides a valuable recruitment and experience-giving function. Institutional myopia, in which only the interests of a closing institution are uppermost, might fail to see this continuing function. This is important because of the prevalence of informal communication within the local labour market.

Such information is not necessarily uni-directional. People may recruit their friends, relatives and spouses but they may also dissuade such others from taking up the work. Concern that such effects are operating to depress general nurse recruitment has already been expressed (Royal College of Nursing 1987). Two aspects of this are important in the present and likely future situations. Firstly, the great reliance of the hospital on informally recruited labour implies a need for the hospital to recognise the value of staff morale for its effects *outside* the organisation. If, as seems to be the case, many (unqualified) staff are working because the job meets a set of requirements which may be difficult to find elsewhere, for example part-time night work, then they will be unlikely to leave when morale declines. If their morale is lowered, however, this might well reduce their incentive to recommend the work to friends. Such negative responses do not incur costs to the person transmitting them. Experience of the client group, even if limited to a short period of service in a declining hospital, is likely to be regarded as a commodity by a community employer. Thus the hospital could also continue to provide a supply fuction to the employment pool as a whole.

Given that we have shown that senior staff with progressive community oriented views are likely to remain with the organisation, their role, as managers, educators and instillers of these views, will probably take on added significance as the hospital runs down. It is especially important that their long term commitment to the client group, and their obvious advocacy of alternative forms of care, should be recognised and understood by those seeking their co-operation in the development of those new forms of care.

5 Job Characteristics

This chapter is concerned with the nature of the job done in the two settings, with the patterns of working of the different categories of staff and their perceptions of the job. We approach the task of characterising the work in several ways. We review the quantitative data that relates to basic job dimensions but we extend that analysis by reference to the qualitative descriptions provided in the interviews or by observation. We repeat this technique with respect to the perceived role.

The organisation of the work

The organisation of work in the two settings differed considerably at the time of our research. The hospital provided 24-hour cover with different sets of people, using a conventional fixed shift system. The community, on the other hand, provided 24-hour cover with the same set of people, using a rotating and flexible shift system. The standard hospital day time cover was provided by staff working two short and two long shifts alternatively, the first running from 7 a.m. to 1.30 p.m., the second from 7 a.m. to 8.30 p.m. As one staff nurse put it

'The long shift enables full planning for the day'

Night cover was provided by staff working a single format shift lasting from 8.15 p.m to 7.15 a.m., thus providing a 15 minute hand-over period at each end. There were two variations to this pattern. A small number of staff, for example, those attached to therapy units, worked fixed daytime hours, while others worked part-time. The latter worked set days or nights. For example, one respondent worked three full nights: Sunday, Monday and Thursday. These patterns had evolved on the basis both of institutional need and individual requirements. Thus the usual pattern was for a person to take whatever shifts (days of the week) were short of staff, and then to try subsequently to arrange for the days of the week that he or she preferred. Most of the people that we spoke to had matched their working arrangements to their personal circumstances in this way.

The situation in the community service was very different; a given person's shifts would vary considerably and would include the 'night shift', termed a 'sleep-in' by the service. As one said,

'Well, for example I'm doing a 10 a.m. to 5 p.m. Monday I'm on 10 a.m. till 7 p.m. and Wednesday from 3 p.m. to 11 p.m., and the sleep-in, and then 7.30 a.m. to 3.30 p.m. on Thursday.'

The basic rate was of approximately three sleep-in shifts per fortnight per person, including the co-ordinators. However, because the sleep-in shift brought an additional allowance, some house co-ordinators would arrange for house companions to do any extra shifts needed to cover for staff absence. Attempts were made to match shift patterns to individual requirements in so far as this was possible. The rota was open to some joint control by staff – in the small scale operation of a single house internal 'covering' was entirely possible. One pattern which had evolved was for 'sleep-ins' to occur in quick succession for staff so that that person could then follow such a period with a longer period of time off. Again, the small scale of the operation required immense flexibility since even single staff absences required quickly arranged cover. The hospital, of course, had a much larger pool of available staff on which to draw in such circumstances. In fact in order to provide flexible cover, the hospital had greatly increased its reliance on 'floating' staff for the night shift.

Quite apart from the total staff/resident ratios, which we reported in Chapter Two, we asked our respondents to tell us how many staff were 'usually on duty' at any one time. Of course cover in the hospital varied according to the severity of need, but the modal response was two (27 per cent). Seventy-nine per cent reported four or less staff on duty at any one time and the average number of residents per unit was 21.2. In the community, the modal response was one (77 per cent) and there were four residents in most of the houses. As Brown and Walton remark (1984, p.222) there is little consistency in the way in which staff-ratios are calculated, but in our view it is the likely number of staff actually expected to be present at any one time which gives the most useful indication.

In practical terms the effects on staff obviously centre around single staff cover. Community staff generally worked on their own. In these circumstances activities which required more than one person could only be provided by shift overlap. The pattern arranged for the houses often allowed only two hours for this (1–3 p.m. usually). To arrange for the weekly staff meeting at one house, for example, two staff would start at 9 a.m. Monday and two at 12 noon or 1 p.m. so that, including the sleep-over person, all five staff would overlap in the middle of that day.

With pressure from staff shortages, either in the establishment or of a temporary nature, there was considerable reliance on overtime working in both organisations. The community staff reported working an average of 2.95 hours overtime in the week prior to our survey, while the hospital staff reported a similar level of 3.5 hours. However, the community staff were much more likely to have done some overtime. In other words overtime was occasionally done by most community staff (88 per cent) but by only about half (57 per cent) of the hospital staff. The reasons for the latter reflect not only the organisation of work in the hospital but also the 'availability' of staff. As we discussed in Chapter Four, staff working in various combinations of shift and part-time arrangements were doing so for domestic reasons. Thus only about a third (36 per cent) of part-time hospital staff ever did overtime, and the average amount of overtime was very different between shifts. Day shift staff had worked an average of four hours in the previous week, night shift staff only 1.5 hours (p<.05).

Similar factors were responsible for voluntary (unpaid) overtime; 86 per cent of those in the hospital who said they occasionally did voluntary work were full time day staff. About a third (36 per cent) of the total hospital staff reported ever doing voluntary work, compared with two thirds (67 per cent) of the community staff. The amount of work involved was also very different. The community staff had worked an average of 3.25 unpaid hours in the week before our survey, the hospital staff an average of 1.85 hours (p<.05).

Work patterns

To try and summarize the work patterns of all our respondents, based on their own reports and our participant and informal observations, was extremely difficult. However, our research was not concerned with evaluation of service provision from the residents' point of view and we did not, for that reason, conduct rigorous observations of staff behaviour. We relied on scales that would abstract the main dimensions of the work and we will turn to those in the next sections. Here, however, we will briefly characterise the main patterns of work in the two settings.

The pace of change, especially in the hospital, made detailed comparisons by unit unlikely to be rewarding. Villas were closing and some of the residents were being moved in groups into villas with characteristically different levels of dependency. Other villas had evolved particular training functions. We decided to include two measures of how staff perceived the general characteristics of the residents. These concerned the degree of dependency, estimated on a three-point scale (low, medium, high) and the proportion of residents with behaviour problems, estimated on a seven-point scale (none, very few, quite a few, half, quite a lot, most, all). These measures were included in order to check overall differences between the organisations and links between these characteristics and staff reactions. In fact both measures produced differences between the organisations which are summarised in Table 5.1. Given the trend reported in Chapter Two, which indicated that the least dependent residents were being discharged first, it is not too surprising to discover that there was more perceived dependency and a greater proportion of behavioural problems in the hospital. Notice, however, that although the overall average was lower in the community on both measures, a single resident exhibiting a major behavioural problem could have a disproportionate effect within the confines of an ordinary house. We shall return to this point later in Chapter Eight.

Table 5.1
Estimated levels of dependency and proportion of behavioural problems

	Community	Hospital	Significance of difference
Dependency score	2.0	2.4	p<.01
Proportion of behavioural problems	1.83	3.34	p<.001

Apart from the specialist departments, and the special needs (behaviour) unit, there were variations in the basic layout of villas, reflecting the fact that some were effectively divided into two units or 'flats' and some were nominally divided into 'ends', by resident capability. In addition there were 'half-way houses' on site where pre-community training was carried on in domestic circumstances. Such training was also increasingly a feature of the work elsewhere, especially in the 'flats'. Some residents attended therapy departments during the day but, amongst the more dependent, the possibility of this could be limited when spare staff were not available to escort them. The pace of change within the institution, reflected in our account at the beginning of this report, meant that changing work patterns were reported by many respondents. Key workers taking over responsibility for doing 'their' residents' laundry on a villa is one excellent example of the way in which the villa was increasing its role as the effective unit within the hospital as a whole.

Within all this variation it seemed best to characterise the general work patterns in two ways: daytime and night time. Although the daytime period was covered by two shifts, all staff would recognise the same pattern across these shifts, except where they changed over from charge nurse to sister. This is because habitual patterns were associated with individuals in charge.

> 'If you're working with sister she'll do the breakfast but she won't help with the bathing ... but the other qualified, they won't start breakfast until all the work's done.'
>
> (Nursing assistant)

Other than these sorts of variations, the daytime pattern was essentially one of routine care tasks, in concentrated bouts, interspersed with quiet periods of much less activity. Typically the day shift started with the hand over, with residents being bathed and dressed from around 7.30 a.m. to 9.15 a.m. Breakfast followed with a medicine round, and a tea break at 11 a.m. After the initial work load, the morning saw the sorting of clothing, laundry and so on and then residents would be made ready for lunch. After lunch there were similar back-up tasks until tea-time around 5.30 p.m. The staff take their late breaks and handover occurs after 8 p.m. The main characteristic of this general pattern was that two periods during the daytime were available for resident interaction of a more directed sort; these occurred in the morning after the support tasks were done, and in the afternoon after lunch was cleared away. These were the periods when staff mentioned specific resident activities. In most cases, the number of residents and staff meant that using routine care tasks as opportunities for training or anything other than basic care was unlikely.

> 'You can't do it really (teach just the one), not when there's all of them to do and just the two of you on' (and on a heavy physically dependent villa) 'you just seem to be giving basic care ... basic care ... you don't get a lot of chance to do anything else with them.'
>
> (Staff nurse)

So if residents did not leave the villa to go to a department, they would only become involved in activities at these times.

The night shift was radically different. The typical pattern here was again dominated by resident ability. Less dependent residents might stay up till 11 p.m. but the highly dependent, physically handicapped people would be got ready and into bed early so that:

'A couple of good nurses, used to lifting, might finish by 11 p.m.'

Because of the general relaxed air in the evening staff tended to describe this as the best time of day. Many reported it as a time when good interaction with residents was possible. Of course, after the evening period the shift was basically one of monitoring the sleeping residents and dealing with any problems that might occur at night.

In the staffed houses of the community service the daily routine also necessarily involved early morning chores and mealtime preparation, but the staff were not doing these 'tasks'. The daily record of activities is a record of supervised resident behaviour. To fit in with the routine of the residents, the staff generally wait for residents to get themselves up and begin breakfast. Chores are shared out, and residents prepare meals in turn. Tasks not yet mastered are treated as opportunities to develop skills and additional skills are taught throughout the day, although each such opportunity may only occupy a short time period:

'There are 28 teachable objectives per day.'

In the evening the residents relax, staff socialise with them, watch TV and, if there are two staff on, maybe take residents out to the pub or to see a film.

The major sources of variation in the routine of the houses are not associated with different shifts of staff but different individuals doing sleep-ins do vary their pattern to a certain extent. Other than personal habits, the major determinant of activity is the presence of more than one staff person. It is this that permits outside 'community' contact.

The working patterns of the different grades of staff also vary to some extent in both settings. As we report later in this chapter, the villa staff tend to work at much the same tasks up to and including charge nurse/sister.

'Even though I'm a ward manager, I have to participate in the routine. It's not only that the work load is high, you have to participate, then the nurses will follow your standard of care.'

In the community service, the co-ordinators also do the sleep-in shifts and 'participate in the routine' but must also supervise staff, attend meetings, work out the rota, do the accounts and so on. The actual pattern varied between the individuals, rather than because of the work role, and, as we report below, despite some feeling that their jobs were mostly about paper work, the house co-ordinators reported a level of resident interaction identical to that of house companions.

The sleep-in shift in the community service differed from the hospital night shift, not only because the staff who did it also worked in the daytime, but also because it was expected that staff would actually sleep throughout the period. When a resident created a disturbance members of staff would be faced with a broken night in the middle of two daytime work periods, although it was possible for staff to phone for support and this had happened on occasion. We shall look at the impact of this and similar problems in Chapter Seven. Now we turn to an examination of these different patterns of work in more strictly comparable terms as we ask 'How did staff characterise their work in terms of its basic dimensions?'

Perceptions of the basic dimensions of the job

There are a number of measures of job characteristics in the occupational literature but the special circumstances of care staff and the work they do required that we amend these and develop suitable questions. We started with the inventory of characteristics developed by Sims et al. (1976) for application to employees in a large medical centre (see Szilagyi et al. 1976). Similar uses have produced consistent results amongst general nurses (Schuler, Aldag and Brief, 1977; Brief and Aldag, 1976; Brief and Aldag, 1978; Lyons, 1971). We then included questions relating to interaction with residents and revised these questions following our pilot work. The final inventory measures six basic dimensions of the work. These are:

Variety of Skills. (abbrev. as Variety) The degree to which staff perform a range of tasks and use a variety of procedures.

Task Identity. (abbrev. Task ID) The extent to which each person can see their own activities as contributing to the complete service provided for residents.

Autonomy. (abbrev. Auton) The extent to which staff are left on their own, to act independently of supervision.

Feedback. (abbrev. Feed) The perceived degree of feedback on job performance.

Interpersonal Interaction. (abbrev. Inter) The extent to which staff interact with people other than residents, especially other staff.

Resident Interaction. (abbrev. Resint) The degree of contact and interaction with individual residents, other than for purposes of basic physical care.

Each question was scored from 1 to 5, from 'very little' to 'a great deal', and there were two questions for each of the above dimensions, so that final values varied between 2 and 10 on each dimension. The questions appear in the appendix, where they are identified by key letters under question 27 of the questionnaire.

The aim of this sort of measure, which is essentially an attributed description, is not merely to provide a numerically expressed map of each job but to help enable us to identify which aspects of the work are in some way critical for the staff. Later in this book we relate the findings on these measures to other individual responses but here our concern is with the overall picture. Three types of observations can be gleaned from the values we obtained. Firstly, we may examine the overall scores, secondly, we may draw profiles of jobs at particular levels and thirdly, we can, of course, make direct comparisons between the hospital and community settings.

It is part of the rationale of scales such as these to provide questions that enable people to respond over a range large enough to allow for detailed comparisons between individuals. Consequently we cannot make much of the overall average scores because they are in part a property of the scale; that is to say we do not know what 'a moderate amount' of, for example, Task Identity means outside of this context. However, when the overall average falls noticeably towards one extreme or the other, we can at least begin to suspect that we have cut across a major feature of the work.

Referring to the original scale values, given at the foot of Figure 5.1, we can see that two of the six dimensions do produce rather extreme results; people tended to attribute fairly high values to Autonomy and fairly low values to Feedback. These two dimensions are reflections of the organisation as well as of the nature of the work. People generally tended to feel that they were left on their own to act independently of supervision, and, in the hospital, this probably reflected the staffing levels and organisation of the work. Identifying low levels of feedback on performance, on the other hand, probably reflects the difficulties people experience in gauging the effect of their efforts, as well as indicating a generally low level of performance review. We will return to these issues as we discuss each dimension in more detail for each particular staff level.

Figure 5.1 shows the profiles of the jobs done by the various groups of staff. In this figure the vertical lines represent the overall average values on each dimension and the lengths of the horizontal bars show the group deviation from this value. In this standardised form the variations shown can be validly compared and statistically tested.

Hospital jobs

If we confine our attention to the hospital staff there are a number of observations that can be made about the overall profiles of each category. The first of these is that the patterns within each grade tend to cohere, that is to say that the changes from grade to grade are generally multi-dimensional and in the same direction. As we move from one group to another, the whole pattern of responses changes. With one or two important exceptions therefore, people are tending to describe noticeably different jobs. Nursing assistants, for example, report lower levels on all dimensions and both groups of qualified nurses report near average levels across most dimensions.

Secondly, we can note that these changes are mostly cumulative through the hospital hierarchy. Although the differences between any two grades may not appear great, and may not in themselves seem large enough to be due to anything but chance, the overall trends are significant. Scores for Variety, Task Identity, Autonomy and Interpersonal Interaction all become larger at higher levels in the hospital hierarchy. This gradual

Figure 5.1

Job profiles of community and hospital staff groups on six dimensions

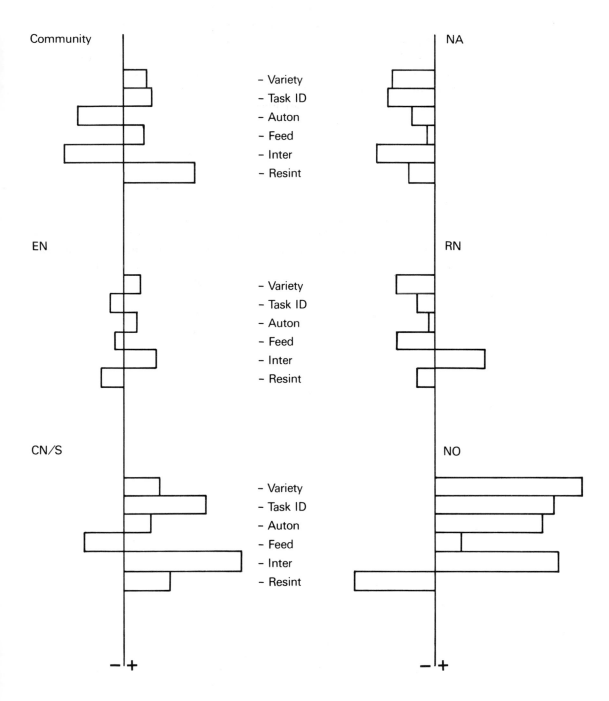

Original scale values for the mean on each dimension:
Variety: 5.57   Task Identity: 5.94   Autonomy: 7.84
Feedback: 4.56   Interpersonal Interaction: 6.13   Resident Interaction: 6.01

increase in the variety and scope of tasks, with greater control and increased interaction with others, is a clear reflection of the hospital hierarchy and the accepted career structure of the occupation. Furthermore, this pattern confirms the validity of our measuring technique. Our main interests, however, must be in noting where the principal changes occur and in identifying particular differences which may signal problems in the organisation.

Whilst the gradual changes we have noted reflect the career structure, the main differences between groups indicate the organisational divide which occurs at the charge nurse/sister level. Figure 5.1 shows that the whole character of the job changes above registered nurse level. This finding would probably seem entirely unremarkable to practitioners in the field. It can also be expressed by saying that the charge nurse/sister role is more like that of the senior nurse than of any other group. However, there is an important and significant deviation from this pattern: the level of Resident Interaction reported by charge nurses/sisters is higher than in any other group. It is not surprising to find that the administrative job of senior nurses is associated with very low levels of reported interaction with residents, but it is less easy to explain why charge nurses/sisters should report levels higher than those of nursing assistants, enrolled nurses and registered nurses.

In order to illuminate these findings, the organisational divide and the pattern of resident interaction, it is necessary to go beyond the basic job profiles and examine the accounts people gave at interview. Following the logic of our approach we were aware of these differences when the interviews were conducted so that we could include questions which covered these areas. There are two main ways in which we analysed the replies to the relevant questions. These were to classify the similarities and differences which people saw between groups of staff and to categorise the kinds of tasks people reported in terms of resident interaction.

On its own, evidence of either the numerical kind, or that based on the interviews, would not be especially compelling but, in fact, the two sorts of information reinforced one another and so helped to explain the major differences we identify above. Firstly, we address the main organisational divide. There are two elements to this; these are the extent to which the apparent similarities of the job below charge/sister level are endorsed by different grades and, secondly, the extent to which the formally defined organisational differences are recognised.

Table 5.2 summarizes our analysis of answers to questions about the differences between qualified and unqualified staff jobs. Naturally such questions contain numerous idiosyncracies and 15 per cent of the replies defied reasonable classification. The three categories given in the table are based on the following logic.

(a)   Larger and wider: qualified staff are attributed work roles which include the tasks of their unqualified colleagues but which also entail more work, responsibility and knowledge of a significant kind.

For example: 'The qualified do all that unqualified do, plus more.' (Charge nurse)

(b)   Responsibility and knowledge: qualified staff are seen as having either a nominal responsibility and/or a specialist knowledge (usually medical) but are attributed roles that are basically the same as the nursing assistants.
For example: 'There are N/As that know as much as me – qualified know about things like petit mal, etc.: and sign forms, but there's no practical difference.' (Enrolled nurse)

(c)   Few differences: these responses minimise the differences between qualified and unqualified staff and, instead, emphasise team working and lack of status differentiation.
For example: 'We all muck in. I know some girls that trained with me – as soon as they're qualified, the power goes to their head.' (Sister)

Table 5.2
Hospital staff descriptions of the nature of qualified staff jobs (per cent of interview responses)

Qualified jobs involve:	CN/S	RN/EN	NA
(a) Larger and wider roles	57	14	6
(b) Greater responsibility and knowledge	29	71	67
(c) Few differences from unqualified jobs	14	14	28

There are two notable features in this pattern of responses and they both reinforce the critical organisational divide. Registered nurses and enrolled nurses reproduce the same pattern as nursing assistants and, significantly, this is a pattern which largely acknowledges the difference between the qualified/unqualified staff but does not emphasise it. Replies in category (b) predominate. The charges/sisters, on the other hand, differ from both groups and typically respond in ways which emphasise the enhanced role of qualified staff.

When people describe the roles of groups other than their own, we learn about the ways in which people place *themselves* in relation to those groups. Here we see the main supervision divide – with registered nurses aligning themselves with their unqualified colleagues. But if people disagree about the most appropriate role descriptions in this revealing way, do they also differ in their views of the formal structure of control?

To answer this, we asked people about autonomy in their work. We knew that there was a general tendency for people to feel that they were left to get on with the job but we also wanted to know what the limits to their decision making were in an organisational sense. In the interviews we asked about six examples of typical decision making at villa level. We were aware that the charge nurse or sister would have the responsibility for these decisions but we also recognised that staff could be more or less involved with, or trusted with, minor operational matters. We asked about buying for residents, ordering repairs, planning holidays and individual programmes and about fixing the staff rota. A convenient way to summarize our findings centres on the staff duty rota. In conditions of staff shortage, which are not uncommon, staff must move to other units at the discretion of the nursing officer. Under normal circumstances, however, the head or acting head of the unit will determine the rota. In practice, each unit tends to run in its own way. Staff shortages often require acting-up, but even when there is a full complement of staff some units share responsibilities below the level of rota control while others refer everything to the charge/sister. Thus the 'rota' tends to represent a limit to the participation of staff. For example:

> 'I always try to involve all staff in all the decisions – especially those concerning residents.'
>
> (Charge nurse)
>
> 'Apart from buying in things, the charge nurse does it all.'
>
> (Nursing assistant)

Table 5.3 shows that the first of these quotations need not be an empty boast; about a third of the responses at all levels agreed that there was some sharing out of minor responsibilities, even if, for example, a signature was required eventually. The second quotation reveals how practice could vary and staff be left with a feeling of only minimal involvement. Where staff felt that participation occurred across the range of items mentioned above we have classified their reply as 'shared up to rota' but where all decisions were apparently passed on by staff to the charge nurse or sister we have classified the reply as 'referred up to rota'.

Table 5.3
Staff accounts of the spread of autonomy within villas (per cent of interview responses)

	CN/S	RN/EN	NA
No real autonomy	—	56	55
Shared up to rota	33	22	27
Referred up to rota	—	11	18
Full unit control	67	11	—

There is a measure of agreement in these estimates in that similar proportions below charge nurse/sister level endorse the pattern given at this level. As we explained earlier in this report, a detailed analysis at unit level was not practicable so we cannot test whether subordinates in particular units agreed on the pattern of responsibilities seen by their charge nurses; since these were openly negotiated issues within units, or accepted customs of practice, it would be strange if there was major disagreement. The important points here are that the formal divide was clear and that the style of control varied in ways that are seen at all levels.

The 'Autonomy' defined by our job inventory can now be seen in its context. Within each unit there was an understanding of the pattern of responsibility – as this worked out in practice rather than as it was bureaucratically defined – and staff were expected to carry on within this framework. Decisions affecting the unit were also limited by routine in that innovations, from whatever source, were referred upwards by charge nurses/sisters.

Although most people reported much the same quite high level of independent working, this narrowly defined 'autonomy' was also seen as limited by accepted routine. As one experienced sister put it:

> 'It's the spur-of-the-moment things you can never do here. The normal things you or I can do, like getting up on a Sunday and saying let's go to the coast. Everything must be planned.'

One of the conclusions of earlier work on organisational structure and care (Raynes, Pratt and Roses, 1979) was that resident-oriented practices were associated with units where staff had some say in decisions about their, largely routine, jobs. We will return to the issue of participation in the next chapter but here we can note that, as one young assistant put it:

> 'The NAs, basically decide what they are going to do, within the unit routine.'

We can add that this pattern is not so much that of the institution, which does have one set of rules, but is rather the ward or unit practice.

So what do staff do, within the constraints of the bureaucracy, that contributes to the variation in levels we have recorded on the other job dimensions? As we made clear at the beginning of this report, it was not part of the research design to evaluate in any detail the care outcomes in either setting. That would have required a longitudinal behavioural analysis which we did not conduct. However, given our various concerns with the skills and experience of staff, it was part of our intention to investigate the conception of the work held by different people, on the assumption that this would tell us both about organisational factors and individual skills.

Of course particular tasks could be expected to vary enormously from ward to ward, and, just as the characteristic decision making pattern operates at ward level so too might the pattern of tasks. Others have reported ward level variations in resident management practices (McLain et al., 1975), and in community care facilities (Bjaanes and Butler, 1974) and in comparisons of both types of service (Rawlings, 1985). Our concern was to identify staff variations that would help provide comparisons between hospital and community. Necessarily, therefore, we must analyse across wards by categories of staff in ways which avoid those particularities. We asked people to describe what they did on a typical day (shift) and included additional questions about specific features of the work. In this analysis, however, our focus must be on the residents, or rather on the way staff relate to residents. We had asked staff to estimate how much resident interaction they experienced. When they described their actual jobs, we could examine how they referred to resident activities and other tasks, in short, how they characterised these interactions and tasks.

Table 5.4 summarizes our analysis of the complete descriptions of daily (shift) work patterns. Naturally people varied in the detail and length of their responses to questions such as these, but we have categorised their job descriptions by type in the following hierarchical manner, noting that individuals in each category may also have made statements similar to those in a more limited category. For example a description placed in group (b) might include both the phrases quoted below in (a) and (b).

(a) Essential care tasks only:
     This group comprises job descriptions that contain no references to interaction with residents at all, or which refer to residents only in respect of basic work routine (eg 'wash and dress them').

(b) Additional interaction:
     Although the example given above might seem to be appropriate here, the distinction we have made centres on the non-essential nature of the interaction or resident centred activity. Residents must be physically cared for, woken up and so on, but additional activities ('getting the jigsaws out') mark a different form of interaction.

(c) More positive interaction:
     The distinction here involves the directedness of the interaction. Any activity can be included as long as it indicates a positive resident-centred task. 'Teaching writing' is a clear example of this kind of task.

(d) Full resident-orientation:
     This category includes those responses which, rather than just mentioning one or more resident centred task, revealed an entirely resident-oriented task structure. Given the hospital organisation, this was unlikely to be a frequent response – though some units do have a philosophy, and claim a practice, based on such a view. (eg 'Our activities here are dictated by individual resident needs').

Table 5.4
Classification of work by the nature of resident interaction (per cent of interview responses)

	CN/S	RN/EN	NA	Total
Essential care tasks only	22	22	41	33
Additional interaction	22	56	41	40
More positive interaction	44	22	18	25
Full resident-orientation	11	—	—	3

The wider and more varied job which charge nurses/sisters describe included more resident interaction, as we noted above. From Table 5.4 it also appears that they typically conceive of the job in a more directly resident oriented manner. Although the overall pattern of responses reflects the basic custodial care model, which would be anticipated in a large hospital, the change at the levels of qualified and senior staff shows how the training they have received, and/or the responsibilities given them, have changed their conception of the work.

At the charge nurse/sister level the more positive orientation that is evidenced here is, as we discussed above, linked to higher reported levels of interaction with residents. Without observational data we cannot confirm the actual pattern of interaction, but it is interesting to note that interaction with others (staff, parents) is also reported as higher at this level. Certainly charge nurses do not seem to believe that their wider jobs, which involve greater dealings with others, preclude their opportunities for active resident interaction. It is the divide between qualified nurses and unqualified assistants that marks the change in interpersonal interactions, and this is a product both of low staffing levels and of the fact that, bureaucratically, qualified staff are usually the ones who must 'deal with others'. Such 'dealing with others' is what produces the high interaction levels amongst senior staff, whereas, for assistants, it is the degree of isolation on the ward that produces the lower level they report.

Table 5.2 showed that registered nurses/enrolled nurses tended to describe their work role in a similar way to nursing assistants. That is to say, both qualified and unqualified staff below charge nurse/sister level minimised the possible differences between themselves and reported 'team working' and 'mucking-in'. From Table 5.4 however, we learn that despite their apparent motivation to reduce any status distinction, qualified staff generally do tend to focus more on the residents.

Again the critical importance of the charge nurse/sister level is emphasised. Their picture of the job is more likely to include activities specially designed for residents. Even when the Individual Care Plans for residents are discussed and implemented by the unit staff it is clear that the charge nurse/sister more often sees the resulting activities as a part of the job. This is encouraging, given that as the hospital population reduces and the proportion of more dependent residents increases, the hospital management continues to press for improvement in care provision. Table 5.4 shows that resident orientation was at higher levels amongst qualified staff in terms of the actual tasks people saw themselves doing, as well as in terms of their patterns of beliefs.

What does not seem to flow downwards, however, is feedback. We cannot make much of the overall low levels reported on our scale, since we lack an appropriate benchmark for judging what 'low' means. The interviews suggested, however, that people felt a genuine lack of information on job performance. The sort of information required varied with the nature of the work, so that the successful completion of basic care tasks and resident objectives might be appropriate for qualified nurses and assistants, while implementing a range of objectives for residents might be seen as appropriate for a sister or charge nurse. Most people, however, were forced to operate on the assumption that only negative feedback was likely.

> 'I get the jobs done, nobody says anything. I'm satisfied, so I carry on until I'm told otherwise.'
>
> (Nursing assistant)
>
> 'I have a job performance review every year from the nursing officer, but it's a paper exercise really.'
>
> (Charge nurse)

Many people also commented on feedback concerning organisational issues and discussion of this will appear in the next chapter. Here we note that the absence of any straightforward technique for judging performance at the operational level is felt by almost all staff.

Community jobs

How did working in the community service compare with working in the hospital? We refer again to Figure 5.1 and note that since community and hospital staff were assessed in the same way, and their responses were standardised to the same overall scale values, the job profiles shown are strictly comparable. It is immediately clear that the community staff described a job that was noticeably different from that described by any group within the hospital. We will comment on each dimension in turn, firstly in terms of the numerical measures and then by reference to the qualitative data.

The community direct care staff reported a level of variety which was essentially no different from most groups within the hospital, excluding the nursing officers. The job seemed to consist of about the same number of different activities for all staff. Task Identity, the extent to which the staff person's efforts seemed to contribute to the whole service, was also near the average. Given the much closer relationship within the houses, and the small complement of staff and residents, this was perhaps a disappointing finding, which showed just how difficult it is for care staff to get a 'complete' feeling for the service.

Autonomy was a different matter. Here we must introduce a distinction between an overall difference and a group difference. Excluding nursing officers, the overall level of Autonomy reported in the hospital was not significantly different from that reported in the community service, but when the separate staff groups were considered, the community staff turned out to report a level of Autonomy which could be statistically bracketed with that of nursing assistants. The house co-ordinators are physically close whenever they are in the house and it may be this closer supervision that is reflected in the lower autonomy experienced by staff. In terms of Feedback community staff were similar to those in the hospital: both groups reported low levels of Feedback. Once again this suggests that staff in both settings found it difficult to know how well, or badly, they performed their jobs.

The next measure in the job profile was Interpersonal Interaction. Here again there was a group similarity: the level of Interpersonal Interaction reported by community staff was statistically similar to that shown for nursing assistants, but in this case there was also a significant overall difference. In other words the community staff reported less Interpersonal Interaction than the average for all direct care staff of the hospital ($p < .05$). Although they were rather more isolated than the average found in the hospital as a whole, therefore, community staff were not significantly more isolated than nursing assistants.

Finally we turn to Resident Interaction. Here again there was an overall difference ($p < .01$) in that community staff reported more such interaction. Since more resident interaction was a main aim of the community service, this finding would seem to be encouraging evidence of some success. It is interesting to note, however, that this higher reported incidence of interaction did not differ significantly from the level reported by charge nurses and sisters.

However, the aim of the staffed housing service is not simply to increase staff/resident interaction, but to change its nature and effects. In the same way, although there may be a similar variety of tasks, these should be a different set from those typical of the hospital. To examine the qualitative differences, we again turn to our interview data, beginning with the issue of Autonomy.

As we noted above the staff rota made a convenient focus for the examination of the extent of autonomy. It was clear that the individual homes constituted the unit in terms of patterns of work, just as the villa did in the hospital. However, although the rota was the responsibility of the house co-ordinator the informal operation of it extended to house companions. The hospital pattern revealed in Table 5.3 is extended by one category in the community, which we could call 'shared up to and including the rota'. One house companion claimed to have no decision making authority, whilst two claimed full unit control. The typical response was either 'referred up to rota' [5] or 'shared up to rota' [6]. This obviously represents rather more shared responsibility than in the hospital, where more than half of staff nurses/registered nurses, enrolled nurses and nursing assistants claimed they had no real autonomy. This raises the question, therefore, of why in the postal questionnaire the community staff reported levels of Autonomy that were statistically much the same as those of nursing assistants in the hospital.

The most likely explanation, and it repeats a theme of this report, was that the expectations of community staff were significantly different from the average within the hospital.

> 'We have a fair bit of say in the house – but not in the service. (So you feel you are directed most of the time?) Oh yes, very much so! (What about the hospital?) Well you didn't *expect* to have much say in the hospital somehow. They kept on about this house that you would run – but you're just a little cog in the wheel.'
>
> (House companion)

As this response illustrates so well, even when the staff acknowledged 'a fair bit of say' they saw the limitations to their autonomy and, given the size of the house and the rationale of the service, they *expected* to have proportionately more authority. In fact, as we discuss in the next section, the staff really did have a considerable input to the house operation and in their accounts they gave plenty of examples of this. It is just that, for many, it is not enough, and this seemed more likely to be a characteristic of them as individuals rather than of the situation itself.

In terms of the tasks which they performed the perceptions of community staff differed from those of the hospital staff. The interview accounts show that the variety of tasks was described as greater than in the hospital. This is unlikely to surprise anyone who has experience in such settings and probably reflects a truly greater diversity in the actual tasks basic care staff do. However, in the postal survey community staff *reported* a level that was not really different from that of most groups in the hospital. Again, it seems likely that this was another reflection of the differing levels of motivation to be found in each organisation. We shall confirm this impression later when we examine satisfaction levels; at this point we note that the variety of tasks runs from high activity to virtually zero during the course of a normal day, in line with residents' requirements. For example:

> 'Often in the evenings we'll just sit and watch telly. We ask the residents but they just seem to want to watch TV. [Is it like a ward then?] No. If they want something we can do it. But I find the evenings really boring. I hate just sitting there and not doing anything. Sometimes I'll just go and clear the kitchen out for something to do.'
>
> (House companion)

Task Identity produced slightly different results. Again the community staff reported a level that did not differ much from the hospital value, but group comparisons showed that the divide between charge nurses and senior nurses on the one hand, and all other hospital grades on the other, also separated community staff. In other words, the latter reported no greater grasp of 'the complete service' than, for example, registered nurses do. Even if one were to argue that this is because the 'service for a resident' might reasonably be interpreted to include aspects of the service provided outside the individual houses, it would not be borne out by the staff's own accounts:

> 'Sometimes I wonder how I fit into the day-to-day running of the house.'
>
> (House companion)

This is partly an organisational point, and partly an interpersonal one. Knowing how and where to 'fit-in' is a function of the planned objectives of the work and the established relationship of the staff person to them. It can also be a function of the relationships established within the unit. Naturally these will vary with the individuals employed but, more generally, we can say the established relationships will depend on the way authority and information are distributed and on the number of people involved. As we have seen, decision making within the houses was well spread, so now we will turn to an examination of the way staff interacted with one another.

Generally, as we noted above, the level of interaction with other staff was lower in the community than in the hospital, although not significantly lower than that experienced by nursing assistants. Much of the time, then, the community staff worked on their own with the residents. When there was an opportunity to interact with other staff this might occur instead of interaction with residents. If, at the same time, there was no immediate programme of activity, or if, for example, the staff were meeting, then the confusion glimpsed in the above quotation increased and the more normal pattern of staff/resident interaction was disrupted. But of course this was not typical of the situation precisely because the usual complement of staff was lower. When only one other person was on duty the resident-oriented activities tended to predominate, especially of course when one person escorted a resident shopping or on a similar outing. It was when the tasks reduced, or when the main routine of the day involved relatively inactive periods, that staff/staff interaction took over.

> [Do you get bored?] 'Yes. If we have tea early – say finished by 7 p.m. Then 7 till 9 p.m. is quite boring. If there is another staff on duty, you tend to talk to that person.'

All of this underlines the need for staff time to be effectively targeted. Inevitably there will be overlaps of duty which will produce little, but generally staff were aware that staff/staff interaction could only predominate when residents themselves choose to ignore them (by watching TV) and that duty overlaps were principally to be seen as opportunities for extra activities with residents.

The only other avenue for interpersonal interaction is with 'the community'. As one house companion put it:

> 'Just about like being a housewife in that way, just when you go shopping or someone calls.'

This, of course, is an incentive to engage in activities that might extend such contact, but, again staff could not leave the house unless there was cover by other staff members. Otherwise the only contacts were with people who called at the house.

> 'The Avon lady came in for a chat the other day. "R" invited her in. But there's not a lot of people call into the house.'

Staff were not overly concerned about this, except in so far as it was limiting for residents and was worse when staff shortage made it difficult to get out. In periods of prolonged shortage, for whatever reasons, staff did report some feelings of isolation. However, to complete the remark made by the companion just quoted:

> 'The residents don't have much contact outside, so they do rely on us. We get to go home.'

Next we turn to the issue of Feedback. We have noted that the 'low' level in the hospital was duplicated in the community. There was little extra that we could learn at interview except that many staff expressed some confusion over the adequacy of their performance.

> 'I passed through my probationary period but I don't know what I've done right or wrong.'
> 'We don't know at all. We do get a review each year which we get to read but that's not much use.'

Clearly it was feedback that was missing, rather than overall performance review, and this was probably a product of the low confidence associated with lack of skills and the lack of clear and available techniques of assessment. The irony was that, in talking about their residents, all the staff said they had seen great changes since the residents had left hospital. However, as this initial change gave way to slower improvement the issue of effectiveness has appeared.

'I know what we're doing is right. I can see it's worked, but you can go a long time before you see a change now. You can't be sure you're doing it the right way.'

One aim of the staffed housing service was to provide an environment and organisation which would permit staff to 'do it the right way'. So, finally, we turn to an examination of the extent to which staff interacted with residents in the community service. The analyses of institutions carried out in the 1970s, which discussed variations between institutions in resident management (eg King et al., 1971) would predict greater proportions of essential care tasks or possibly 'Additional interaction', to use our category titles from Table 5.4, in the hospital. Amongst community staff, who reported a significantly higher level of interaction, few described their jobs in these terms.

When community staff described a typical day's work, 35 per cent of their descriptions could be classified as being based on 'More Positive Interaction' and sixty-five per cent as exemplifying 'Full Resident Orientation'. This is very different from the pattern of responses obtained in the hospital, and summarized in Table 5.4. Interestingly the proportion of community staff classified under the heading of 'More Positive Interaction' was very similar to that for charge nurses/sisters. In the community, however, it was the house companions who produced that kind of description. All the co-ordinators we spoke to made statements which were subsequently classified under the heading of 'Full Resident Orientation'. Although this difference could be due to chance, statistically speaking, it follows the pattern shown in Table 5.4 in that the more senior staff reflected the more complex view of the occupation in a way which was entirely consistent with the professional nature of their jobs.

So far we have not differentiated between house companions and house co-ordinators. Their jobs are different, of course, given their managerial function but co-ordinators do sleep-in shifts like companions, as well as paperwork, so that their jobs are a mix of resident centred and bureaucratic tasks, as is the case for charge nurses/sisters in the hospital.

With respect to the job dimensions we have discussed there were no statistical differences between house co-ordinators and house companions. Even in the critical case of Resident Interaction, which co-ordinators typically saw in terms of a 'Full Resident Orientation', the *levels* of interaction were exactly the same between companions and co-ordinators. This represents another difference between the two organisations. In the hospital, the level of ward management was characterised by a major change in the reported nature of the job. Clearly, in the community, even though co-ordinators do a range of bureaucratic tasks that companions generally do not do, this has not led them to move away from their commitment to resident-centredness.

The higher level and different quality of resident interaction evidenced by these replies is a vindication of the belief that care in the community would work in this way. Though only 35 per cent of staff had qualifications in mental handicap, 47 per cent had had hospital experience. This underlines the fact that appropriate changes in organisations can result in very different patterns of care, as Tizard et al. (1975) argued, but raises again the issue of staff competence. Having the right sort of orientation is perhaps a good start, but various constraints and lack of training will limit the next most important factor, namely the contribution of the individual in the professional sense. We have traced a certain confusion in the vision staff have of their contribution to the complete service, and remarked on their sense of a lack of performance feedback. The next stage, therefore, is to ask in a more direct way about staff perceptions of their professional role.

Perceptions of work roles   In order to complete our examination of individuals' perceptions of the job we need to adjust our focus to encompass the whole of the role that staff are asked to fill in the two organisations. Thus we need measures which go beyond simple estimates of the amount of any one dimension on the job. Rather we need to estimate the degree to which individuals understand and concur with the goals of the employing organisation. Clearly, measures of this kind bridge the gap between individuals' characteristics and the properties of the organisation.

Role theory was developed within social psychology to provide a framework which could bridge these properties (Katz and Kahn, 1966; Kahn et al., 1964) and the measures of Ambiguity and Conflict have proved useful in a variety of studies. Significantly lower levels of these aspects of the work role have been found to be related to improved satisfaction and reduced absenteeism amongst nurses (Gray-Toft and Anderson, 1985).

We employed two scales first developed by Rizzo et al. (1970) and extensively tested on a number of samples including nursing personnel (Seybolt and Pavett, 1979; Shuler, Aldag and Brief, 1977; Szilagyi, 1977). The first of these, Role Ambiguity, concerns the extent to which employees are aware of what is required of them by the organisation and is measured by the sum of responses to the first six statements of question 28 on the questionnaire. These statements cover ambiguity over authority, goals and task aspects of the work. The second scale, Role Conflict, concerns the extent to which employees are experiencing contradictory demands, either because the organisation asks them to comply with two or more incompatible requests, or because the organisation requires them to carry out activities with which they personally disagree (eg Redfern and Spurgeon, 1980). It is measured by the sum of the scores on the remaining eight statements of question 28.

This latter point is particularly salient in the context of professional or semi-professional work. The issue of professional conflict with organisational bureaucracy has a long history in the literature (Corwin, 1961) but recently the notion that such conflict is in some sense necessary or inevitable has been challenged (Davies, 1983). The point made by Davies is that institutions not only provide an important reward structure for professionals, but that they also change dynamically in response to demands, which can include 'professional values'. The present case constitutes an example of this, in that the community service provided a radically different organisation facilitating different professional practice, whilst the hospital continued to operate within the established framework.

Both role measures present statements which staff are asked to judge on a scale scored from 'very false' (value 1) to 'very true' (value 7). Ambiguity consists of six statements, giving a possible range of 6 to 42, and Conflict consists of eight statements, giving a range of 8 to 56. The Ambiguity scale was rescored so that high values represent greater Ambiguity.

How do the perceived roles of the different staff groups within the hospital vary, and in what ways do the community and hospital staff differ? Figure 5.2 shows the values obtained on these two measures for each of the hospital staff groups, standardised, as in the previous diagram, on the overall average values so that the groups are comparable statistically. More Ambiguity and greater Role Conflict are shown by bars to the right of the vertical line which represents the overall average.

Figure 5.2

Role ambiguity and conflict expressed by community and different grades of hospital staff

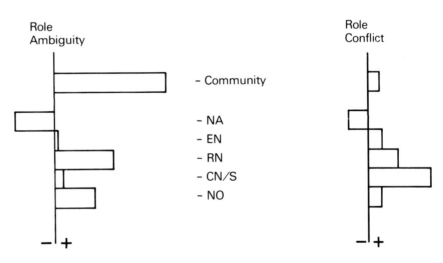

Note: bars to the right of the vertical lines indicate:
a) more role ambiguity
b) more role conflict

We shall comment initially on the hospital staff. There are two observations which can be made. Firstly, we can note that for both scales there appears to be a gradual increase as we move up the established hospital hierarchy. This is perhaps especially noticeable in the case of Role Conflict, but in both cases this 'linear trend' was confirmed by statistical testing (p < .01). In other words the more senior staff experience progressively more ambiguity in their defined roles and felt increasing degrees of conflict. It was nursing assistants, in both cases, who scored lowest; they had the most clearly defined roles and they experienced the least conflict between their conception of those roles and their views of what was expected of them.

The second thing we may note is that there are no large anomalies in the pattern for Role Conflict, although, in the case of Role Ambiguity, the value obtained from staff nurses was significantly higher than that of nursing assistants. In other words the gradual shift in ambiguity revealed by the linear trend is largest across what is approximately the professional divide. This sort of finding is consistent, of course, with the notion of professional working being to some extent in conflict with institutional requirements, which we discussed above. In this case the professional divide was more clearly seen in the case of Role Ambiguity, whilst the highest level of Role Conflict was reported by charge nurses/sisters and emphasised their intermediate managerial position.

What light can we throw on these findings from our observations and interviews in the hospital? The single most important issue was that of staffing levels. This was one of the items in the Conflict scale and it produced the highest mean value (4.5). The topic was mentioned by many of those whom we interviewed and was referred to as the 'never ending problem of the service' by one nursing officer. As we showed in Chapter Two, the nurse-resident ratio has improved historically but people who had known the crowded wards of the past were also aware that new programmes and care plans were difficult to implement whilst staffing remained at the minimum necessary for a custodial style of care. The move to the community, which has left a higher proportion of more dependent residents in hospital, has increased the difficulties for staff trying to improve care. Even escorting a resident to the therapy centre was problematic if there was no one spare in the villa. The shortage resulted in staff being asked to move to other villas to provide minimum cover so that even when there were higher numbers most staff expected one of their number to be removed. However, what may be seen as a nuisance or even as a neutral aspect of the job for nursing assistants was clearly a source of role conflict for those with the responsibility to arrange staffing levels operation-ally. Our analysis showed that this item differentiated between qualified and unqualified levels, with charge nurses, for example, expressing much greater conflict by scoring 5.6 against the overall average of 4.5 ($p < .01$).

What other aspects of conflict contributed to the overall trend towards greater conflict in the senior levels of the hierarchy? Essentially they were bureaucratic aspects, as might be expected. 'Rule bending', 'inadequate resources' and 'unnecessary tasks', were all significantly more likely to be mentioned at the charge nurse/sister level, as opposed to the nursing assistant level. Here then is a picture of struggle focusing on villa management. We will examine the organisational aspects of this in the next chapter; here we concentrate on the ways in which perceptions of the role are affected by particular aspects of the job.

'Getting the job done' at the level of the villa often seemed to consist of 'getting the staff for the job'. But there was also a Catch-22: as responsibility was spread downwards by the absence of senior personnel, the operational staff must 'act-up'. These temporary changes or extensions to role were added sources of stress for some people, but it was not just the extra burden that caused conflict.

> 'If you're on your own, having been moved somewhere with which you are unfamiliar, and something goes wrong, you are held responsible. Then they turn round and say "why didn't you ask for help" – well obviously they've got no help to give you!'
>
> (Acting charge nurse)

What about the more 'professional' aspects? As we have shown, the charge nurses/sisters, and to a lesser extent the other qualified staff nurses, tended to describe their jobs in ways which revealed more resident-centred activities. Obviously the scope for such activities was limited by the staffing problem and this was a typical response from interviewees who mentioned staff shortages. At the same time Individual Care Plans and Community Skills Teaching were being introduced, so that increased role conflict seemed a likely outcome of the changes in the service. This underlines another theme of this report, which is that the closure of the hospital must not simply consist of a process of reduction at all costs. If staff experience greater conflict as the process continues, they may exacerbate problems by reducing their commitment to resident-oriented care, in order to cope with the increased bureaucratic demands, or they may absent themselves and so add to the problem of staffing levels.

To what extent were Role Ambiguity and Role Conflict experienced by staff in community service? The first thing to note is that the two aspects of role produced very different findings. When we made an overall comparison between staff in the two settings (excluding senior nurses) there was greater Ambiguity to be found in the community ($p < .001$) but essentially the same level of Role Conflict. The difference in Ambiguity was systematic, that is, it occurred on all but one item on the scale, item 2, which reads 'Clear, planned goals and objectives exist for my job'. The fact that *no* two groups varied in their response to this item is revealing. People generally, in both organisations, were aware of the existence of organisational goals, but when it came to how they fitted into the scheme for obtaining those goals, confusion appeared. In the hospital, the differences on other operational items tended to reflect the professional divide, as we noted. What is interesting here is that the community staff, who included many who were unqualified, reported a situation that required a higher level of professional input. This was clearly a reflection of two features of their jobs. Firstly, there is the inappropriateness of highly structured or detailed supervision in the staffed houses, which would have been perceived as an unwarranted increase in the 'institutional' nature of the service. Secondly, it is a straightforward reflection of a lack of training in a range of skills. Lacking such supervision and without adequate training, it is no surprise that community staff were rather less sure about what was expected of them. It is also interesting to note that anticipation of this difference was one response of hospital staff to the possibility of community employment.

> 'Well, the job is not easy and it is easy. It's hard because ... you've got so much to do, you've got no backup and all this ... and you've got to get this done and that done ... It's hard in that way but it's easy in the fact that you don't often have to think. After you've been here so long it's mechanical. But in the community I should imagine it's a lot more thinking.'
>
> (Enrolled nurse)

It is worth adding that this particular respondent was actively seeking a job in the community herself. Thus the increase in Role Ambiguity in the community need not be seen as a negative finding, since a moderate degree of ambiguity and conflict may reflect the broader professional role that the job may offer. The size of the difference suggests, however, that the lack of training in the community was problematic for staff. The feelings of ambiguity expressed here reflect a lack of confidence that can only be improved by training, since increased bureaucratic control is seen as self-defeating.

In this respect the level of Role Conflict is also revealing. Being no different from that found amongst hospital staff it suggests that the existing organisational demands on individuals had not reduced. Of course it is possible that the rather different personnel of the community service, being highly motivated, had lower thresholds for perceiving possible conflict with the hierarchy. To get at the possible factors behind this finding we also asked community staff about problems with the organisation. It became clear that house level organisation meant that conflict was seen as coming from above, from the service management, or, more usually, from local authority requirements.

> 'A lot of the time when I should refer things I don't, just purely because of the aggravation.
>
> (House co-ordinator)

Within the community service there was a tendency for feelings to 'even out' in a way which suggested that the main divide was that between houses and management. In the hospital professional qualifications marked a crucial divide in terms of ambiguity, while conflict reflected the organisational divide at villa level. In the community it seemed that distant bureaucratic requirements were seen by staff as interfering more directly in their professional view of how the service should be run. We will examine these organisational factors at greater length in the next chapter.

6   Organisational Factors

This chapter concerns the way staff saw their employing organisations and their union or professional organisation. At the end of Chapter Five we examined the ways in which staff saw themselves in relation to the organisational roles they occupied. In this chapter, we turn first to a direct examination of how staff perceive the organisation itself, and then go on to discuss their views on supervision and management. We review the management of closure in terms of staff morale. Finally we discuss differences in staff representation.

Perceptions of the organisation

In their study of organisational structure and care practices in the field of mental handicap, Raynes et al. (1979) drew on an earlier tradition of research into aspects of organisational control and employee response that highlighted the importance of individual motivation. They reviewed the studies that had suggested links between centralisation, defined as delegation of authority, and resident orientation (Holland, 1973; King et al. 1971). In the original work on centralisation (Aiken and Hage, 1966, Hage and Aiken, 1967) the authors had identified heirarchy of authority, defined as delegation, and participation in decision making, as the two major components.

One thing that was clear in the initial stages of our study was that the two organisations we were to examine had very different control hierarchies. Indeed, the community service was designed in part on the basis of the approach that had grown from the findings of previous research. To quote Raynes et al.

> 'We have repeatedly shown that decentralisation of authority, that is the involvement in decision making of both direct-care workers and their immediate supervisors, the building heads, had positive consequences for the care of residents' (p.157)

As a first step in measuring responses to the organisations, therefore, we decided to include measures of perceived Hierarchy of Authority and Participation in Decision making. As with our other measures, these would help us to make comparisons between the two settings and between seniority groups within organisations. Rather than extending the comparisons made in the literature between structure and resident care, which we could not independently assess, our aim was to identify the perceived loci of organisational authority and the problems associated with them. (c.f. Pierce and

Dunham, 1978; Pierce et al. 1979). Perceived Hierarchy of Authority was measured by the sum of responses to the first five statements of question 30, which concern the passing of decisions to higher levels of authority. Participation in Decision making was measured by the sum of responses to the final four statements of question 30.

Figure 6.1

Perceptions of the degree of hierarchy of authority and participation in decisions for community and different grades of hospital staff.

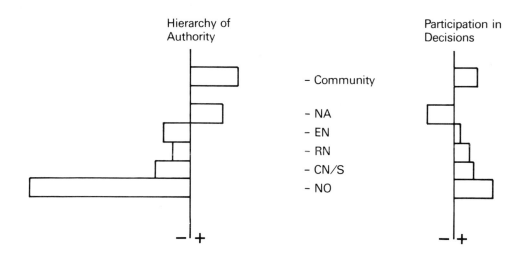

Note: Bars to the right of the vertical lines indicate that:
a) staff perceive a greater degree of hierarchy
b) staff feel others participate more in decision making

Figure 6.1 shows the results obtained from these two measures, broken down by staff groups. In each case the community staff are shown on the same scale, which is standardised to the overall average represented by the vertical line. Bars to the right indicate more than average amounts. There was no significant difference between house co-ordinators and house companions within the staffed houses so all community staff responses are represented by one bar in the diagram.

Firstly, we will consider the findings within the hospital. As would be expected, given the nature of these measures, there is a pronounced effect associated with the actual hierarchy in the hospital. It is clear when looking at Figure 6.1 that the amount of perceived heirarchy decreases as the seniority of staff increases. The nursing assistants see the greatest Hierarchy of Authority and the nursing officers see the least. (This overall trend is highly significant statistically (p<.001). Similarly there is a tendency for Participation in Decision Making to increase with seniority (p<.05). However, although such findings reflect the validity of the measures, they are much less interesting than the group differences. For example, the overall

71

trend of the Participation measure is not marked by any great discontinuities. The gradually increasing amount of perceived Participation in Decision-making reflects what those in more senior positions actually experience. In the case of Hierarchy, however, the questions refer more to the actual approval of decisions, rather than some level of participation in making them. Here there is a major difference between the senior nurses (including directors) and all other grades (p < .05). This, of course, is different from the major divide, reported in the last chapter, between the charge nurse/sister level and nursing officers on the one hand and registered nurses, enrolled nurses and nursing assistants on the other. With the obvious exceptions of Resident Interaction and Autonomy, that divide occurred at the level of villa management, whilst the experience of Role Ambiguity divided across the professional boundary and the degree of Role Conflict also peaked at villa management level. The essentially similar values for Hierarchy reported by all groups below the senior level confirm the extent to which the bureaucratic divide isolates the villas.

When we asked about problems in the organisation it was often operational decisions across this divide that came up. The same kind of complaints came from nursing assistants and sisters about, for example, minor purchases needing written authorisation. As the pressure for improved conditions on the villas builds up, the staff tend to respond with frustration over those occasions when their atttempts to 'personalise' residents' property are seen to be thwarted by decisions made across this managerial boundary. It was in recognition of the central importance of the villa level that the incoming Unit Manager replaced the dual charge nurse/sister grades with a single villa manager. Clearly to improve the efficiency of the villa operation requires the devolution of as much operational authority as possible to this level. We shall return to this issue when we discuss management more generally below.

In the hospital our study documented a structure that is probably well understood by senior management, but it was not our intention merely to provide a description of what may already be known in the service. Rather we thought to present a rigorous means of comparing two very different settings. It turned out that the degree of Hierarchy of Authority and the preceived degree of Participation in Decision making reported by community staff were not substantially different from those reported in the hospital. A statistical comparison between the community staff and the direct care staff of the hospital revealed that there were no real differences in these scores.

The organisation of the community service, and its management philosophy, would suggest that if not the actual decision making hierarchy, then at least the participative bias in decision making should produce an effect on such measures. In fact, although the level of participation reported is the same as that for qualified staff in the hospital, the difference visible in Figure 6.1 between these groups and, say, nursing assistants, is not large enough to be due to anything but chance.

Of course the actual nature of the two organisations was rather different, so it was at least possible that the type of decisions thought to be limited, and the extent of the hierarchy, were also different from those typical of the hospital operation. In our interviews we asked about problems in the organisation. We also followed up such questions with further enquiries about the parties thought to be responsible, but framed this as a neutral question (eg what is responsible for that?). Many of the answers were unique and, in addition there were several people who could not adequately reply. Of the hospital replies we were able to classify sixty-six per cent, of the community replies seventy-six per cent. The categories are slightly different and are given in Table 6.1.

Table 6.1
Perceived problems and attribution of responsibility in hospital and community services (per cent of classified responses)

	Problems		Responsibility for problems	
	Hospital	Community	Hospital	Community
Organisational (eg shifts)	48	54	19	—
Management	37	—	46	92
Residents	11	23	4	—
Professional	—	23	—	—
Policies	—	—	12	—
Personalities	—	—	—	8
No responsibility identified	—	—	19	—

Half the problems mentioned were organisational or operational, such as shifts leading to unfinished jobs or inadequate staffing levels. In the hospital, a sizeable proportion of problems were associated with the management, and were either bureaucratic problems such as excessive paperwork, or other management requirements which caused trouble. In the community, no problems were directly attributed to the management structure in this way. Problems tended to be interpreted as professional disagreements. The picture was very different for the classification of attributed responsibility. Much of the blame in the hospital, even for management-related problems, was seen in a rather neutral way. Although nearly half the responses did attribute responsibility to the management, the other half of the hospital responses emphasised difficulties in actually doing the job, or were refusals to allocate responsibility altogether. Almost all the community responses identified the management as the source of problems. In two thirds of cases the problems took the form of a dispute between a particular house and the project management, but some were between the house and the more distant local authority bureaucracy, while a minority consisted of disputes between a house co-ordinator and the house companions.

There would seem to be two ways in which to account for the differences between the hospital and the community. Either the scale of the hospital produces more complex organisational problems, which are a property of the system itself or, more likely, the scale of the hospital makes responsibility less easily identifiable. The new structure brought in just after our interviews not only introduced single villa managers but also reduced the number of senior nurses. Our results tend to endorse the philosophy of the manager who brought in these changes, in that the real and apparent diffusion of responsibility will have been reduced by such changes.

In the community, the comparison is stark. The smaller scale and simpler structure meant that almost all problems were attributed to a mangerial source. For example, in the hospital if the residents were seen as responsible for a problem, or were described as a problem, then that was the explanation in itself. In the community if a resident or group of residents was a problem, then that was 'the management's fault' for allocating that resident to that house or to that staff person or whatever. This is not too surprising a finding. The rationale of small units is partly about the devolution of responsibility. Such a process means that 'problems' are unlikely to be defined in ways which implicate the small unit itself. Except in the case of 'personality' most people would attribute such a 'problem' to an outside cause. In the hospital many other causes can be thought up.

This highlights the need for the confidence that only training and/or experience can provide, since the community management must turn many such problems down again, to the house level, as the effective unit. A similar process might well be anticipated in the hospital, as the responsibility at villa level has been concentrated and increased. There is a clear message here for hospital villa management support. The previous system, and the traditional pattern in the recent historical past, has been one of 'administration'. The move towards more direct management will concentrate attributed responsibility, so that villa managers will face increased pressure from staff. This has important implications for training at this level, as we shall discuss in Chapter Eight.

However, many of the issues which arose in both settings, even quite minor operational ones, could be thought of as the consequences of 'policy' rather than management. Alternatively they could be linked to decisions at entirely different levels and beyond the immediate institution. As we noted, some community staff placed responsibility for problems at a level above their immediate service managers. So we could ask in a more general way how each of the various main levels of the two organisations were viewed in terms of their responsibility for problems. Such a question is partly about loyalty but it is also about effectiveness. In the case of the hospital, for example, it will be more difficult for local management to manage the crises of morale associated with closure if the main responsibility for 'morale problems' is seen by the staff to lie at some higher level. In other words, this is also a communication issue.

We thus decided to ask staff which levels of the complete organisation had what levels of responsibility for a range of problems. We wished to ask this in such a way that we could properly deduce the relative attributed effect of each level. In order to do this we asked staff to rank four levels of organisational authority in terms of their contribution to problems of morale and the provision of effective care. Using an established method for scaling rankings into measurable intervals, we counted the number of times each level of authority appeared at each rank, in order to indicate its relative importance (Torgerson, 1958). In other words we derived a scale of authority which showed not only the rank of each level but its relative responsibility for attributed problems translated into distances between points. The results are displayed in Figure 6.2. The distances between the points on each line are a direct measure of how much more responsibility for problems the staff thought each level had. Greater responsibility is shown to the right of the mid point, lesser to the left.

Figure 6.2 shows that the rank order matches the formally defined hierarchy, with one anomaly. We included the 'Government' because it seemed possible that staff might simply want to attribute blame to a most distant authority, but although it scored highest amongst community staff, just above the local authority level, it got little more blame than local management in the hospital. Otherwise the hospital staff reproduced the authority structure of the NHS in a conventional manner.

Figure 6.2

The perceived relative responsibility for low morale of different levels in the authority structure of the two services.

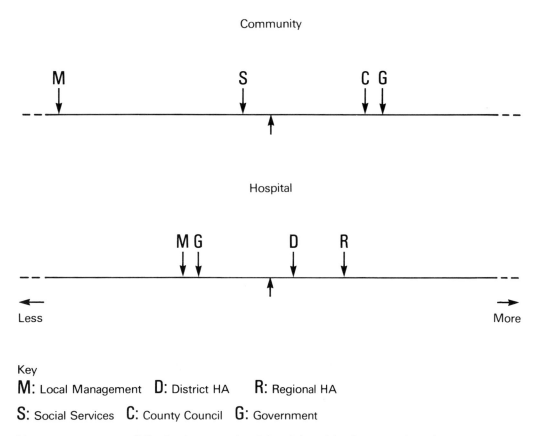

Key

M: Local Management   **D**: District HA   **R**: Regional HA

S: Social Services   **C**: County Council   **G**: Government

Note: greater responsibility is shown to the right of the mid-point on each scale

Two important features of the situation were revealed by this analysis. The first was that the total 'bureaucratic range' seen in the community service was twice as large as that in the hospital. The second was that the relative contribution of the two higher levels (ignoring Government) was different. Specifically, staff in the community tended to see an approximately equal separation between Area Social Services and the County Council, whereas staff in the hospital tended to see only about half the separation between Region and District as between District and local management.

What do we learn from this analysis? The main thing perhaps is that although the ordering reproduces the conventional authority structure, it could have been the exact reverse, in that local management could have been seen as most responsible for low morale. Occasional comments and casual observation might well have endorsed such a view, but it was clear from the findings that staff generally recognised the greater responsibility of higher management. It is also clear that the community service blamed its management relatively less than the hospital staff blamed its, or, conversely, that the community staff blamed the County Council relatively more than hospital staff blamed the Region.

One way in which to describe these findings is to see the overall pattern as a map of the authority structure, seen from below. As we mentioned, the smaller separation of the two levels above the hospital makes the distinction between them less clear. The hospital staff tended to bracket the District with the Region as joint agents of uncertainty. This pattern was the same across four of the five items in this question (question 40), except in the case of the item worded 'bringing about low morale', where the respective ranks of Region and District were reversed and District attracted most blame. By contrast the Area Social Services and the County Council were much more clearly separated by community staff. These different understandings almost certainly reflect the experiences of staff, and their exposure to statements of various kinds from their respective managements. For example, community staff were aware of the nature of Local Authority input simply because some of the routine operation of the service originated at that level. They experienced its remoteness when anything went wrong with their pay, which came from the distant Treasurer's deparment. They had been delayed in the beginning, waiting for houses which were subject to planning permission for 'change of use'. At the time of the research, even the houses' service bills (gas and electricity) were paid at County Council level. Within the houses many routine matters, some of which were formally the responsibility of house co-ordinators, were understood by most staff. As we have shown, only a minority of staff traced management-related problems to disputes within the community houses. In other words the house was the effective unit. Whereas in the hospital disputes over operational issues tended to be seen as between the villa and hospital management, in the community difficulties with the County Council bureaucracy were encountered directly at house level. This would seem to indicate some confusion over the level of effective control which the Local Authority had thought appropriate to vest in the operational unit.

A member of the hospital staff commented 'management is the fashionable word', but clearly the re-organisation of the health service, and the re-structuring of the area social services, was already leading, during the period under study, to a much more visible and positive style of decision making. The Griffiths Report (1983) recommended greater clarification of roles and an increase in delegation. The revised organisational structure we described in Chapter Two clearly reflected these ideas, with the single villa management level. However, the range of decisions taken at this level had not greatly increased. In the community the houses already had considerable decision-making power and were arguing for more. The model of care employed by the community service stressed that residents' own autonomy should be progressively increased in line with their developing abilities. This meant that unless, for example, the purchase of ordinary household items could be decided at house level, the potential for teaching normal responsibilities would be thwarted.

We wondered how house co-ordinators, who had the main operational responsibility for the individual houses, felt about their levels of responsibility. Whilst there was agreement that major budget items should normally be referred upwards, there was some frustration at the system in use, and the detailed budgeting requirements. However, house co-ordinators considered that their level of authority, as defined by their grading, did not warrant full control of the household budget. The increased responsibility would have to be reflected in terms of their salaries and career grading. Delegating larger financial decisions to house level would fit in the with the ideals of the service and could be more efficient, but it would impose greater burdens on house co-ordinators.

We also asked about the other services used by the community houses. Being in the community meant using the local general practitioner, dentist and community speech therapist and the services of the occupational therapy and psychology departments, as well as adult education and all the normal provisions of the local area. Staff reported very few problems in the utilisation of such services, other than one or two problems with general practitioners and a shortage of speech therapy. Access to local facilities was the concern of all members of staff in the community, since all were involved in the running of the houses in a way that was very different from that which was expected of basic care staff in the hospital.

Support to staff

At the beginning of this chapter, we looked upwards at the organisation and examined the way in which staff allocated responsibility for morale and for problems within the organisation. We now turn to the supervision and support which flowed downwards from managers to staff at lower levels. How adequate were supervision and support? We have three sources of information which are relevant to this question: an item from the job satisfaction questionnaire concerning management and supervision; three sets of questions relating to support; and the replies in the interviews to neutrally worded questions about support.

At this point we interpolate a brief note about support. We were dissatisfied with our operationalisation of this concept for two reasons. There is some evidence for the value of interpersonal variables in predicting nurses' reactions (Decker, 1985) and for the role of supervision variables (Sheridan and Vredenburgh, 1978), but we wished to relate support to various levels within each organisation. Only one measure in the literature seemed suitable (Caplan, 1971) since it distinguished between sources of social support originating with subordinates, peers and superiors. In our questionnaire we used three pairs of questions relating to these levels, each scored to produce three scales taking values in the range from 2 to 10. The scales relating to peers and subordinates produced very little variation between groups. The questions seemed to be interpreted as being about loyalty and the answers suggested that whatever support people did experience it was across the main supervisory divide that the biggest effects were to be found. Subsequently we can clarify what we think is a confusing word, much used in the services we examined, by recognising three dimensions in the concept of support. We offer the following classification: support can comprise

(a)   resources (the ability to supply resources, including professional advice and training)
(b)   representation (managerial or 'political' backing)
(c)   socio-emotional aid (befriending, stress-reduction) (Fusilier et al. 1986)

We conceive of these as independent so they can be present to different degrees in different ways. For example, managers might be in a position to provide (a) and (b), but not (c), whilst supervisors might be able to provide (b) and (c). Given that this conception grew out of our research, we could not build this concept into the work at an early stage; thus our discussion of support in the two organisations is necessarily simplified. Our classification, however, helps us to explain what might otherwise appear as anomalous results.

Our first measure of support, which was concerned with satisfaction with 'management and supervision', produced no significant differences, either between the hospital and the community, or between the different grades within the hospital. In terms of support received from supervisors, there were clear differences between grades of staff, with higher grades feeling that they received less support ($p < .01$). We would now characterise this measure as largely concerned with types (b) and (c) support. There was a particularly sharp discontinuity between the levels of villa management (charge nurses and sisters) and nursing officers. This discontinuity was also unlikely to be a chance effect ($p < .05$) and was yet another indication of the crucial importance of villa level in the organisation.

The interviews produced information about two different aspects of support; these were the degree of support that individuals experienced and the sources of that support. Given the considerable variations in the meaning of this term only a coarse categorisation seemed appropriate for degree of support. Table 6.2 accordingly sets out a two-way measure of sufficiency of support as perceived by the different grades of staff.

Figure 6.3

Amount of perceived support received from immediate supervisor

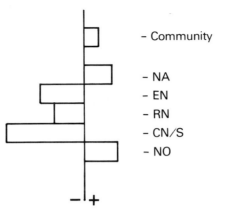

- Community
- NA
- EN
- RN
- CN/S
- NO

– | +

Note: Bars to the right of the vertical line indicate greater support

Table 6.2
Sufficiency of support received by community and different grades of hospital staff (per cent)

	Community	C/N or sister	Other qualified	Assistants
Insufficient support	70.6	77.8	66.7	18.2
Sufficient support	29.4	22.2	33.3	81.8

(The differences are not due to chance: $p < .001$)

House co-ordinators were included in the community category. All of them claimed insufficient support. Taking the house companions alone showed that 64 per cent claimed insufficient support, so the pattern is consistent with the suggestion that it was only the hospital nursing assistants who perceived little need for additional support.

This is a very large difference and shows that some lack of support was reported by all qualified staff in the hospital. As we showed in the previous chapter, nursing assistants, who of course comprised the great bulk of the hospital staff, described jobs which were narrower in content, more isolated but better defined. By contrast the qualified staff experienced greater ambiguity in their broader jobs. The uncertainties of the work role, and their greater responsibilities, generated greater needs for support (especially of types (b) and (c)). This trend culminated in a significant divide at villa management level.

These data were collected before the re-organisation took place. Each villa was essentially covered by one of two shift managers. Now only one person has that responsibility and for 24-hours on call. Already, before the re-organisation, it was clear that many staff at the charge nurse/sister level found the job a strain. Pressure in such positions came both from above and below and some were ill prepared for the role:

'Acting-up is a problem (Why?)'
'It's a strain. Suddenly everybody wants something from you.'
(Charge nurse)

Clearly, with the increase in responsibility represented by the concentration of authority in one person, preparation for and support in the role will be important. Support in the form of representation or 'backing for decisions' seemed to be present when dealing with, for example, the doctor, but what we have called type (c) support was often seen as missing.

'The nursing officer is there to back you up, but being 'managers' seems to mean that they don't need to come out of their office'.

Those who had done their job as part of the former administrative organisation had not yet understood that the new version of 'management' involved a greater responsibility at each level, and it was not surprising to discover that training in management was felt to be lacking by those facing this situation, as we shall show in Chapter Eight.

House co-ordinators identified a similar lack. They spoke of the need to 'seek support' or said simply that they were 'not supported at all, but left to get on with it.' There were two aspects to this situation. Training in management skills is one to which we have already referred, but there was also an organisational reason for the apparent isolation of the co-ordinators at the time of our interviews. As the scale of the new service increased, the single management team was quickly and greatly stretched. An intermediate post has subsequently been created, but in the early stages of the service the only support that co-ordinators could expect was from the central management team. Typically that support was more related to immediate resource needs than anything else. Assistance in dealing with episodes of challenging behaviour from some residents and other similar professional input, as well as arranging for cover when staff numbers were temporarily lowered by absence, was provided from the centre. Although such crisis management was entirely necessary, it carried an ambiguous message. Attribution theory (Jones and Nisbett, 1971) would suggest that house staff and management were likely to interpret these situations differently. Even though the staff requested assistance, the act of assistance could be interpreted as a lack of confidence in their (the staff's) abilities. Similar evaluations are known to occur in the other direction, when supervisors attribute lack of ability as a result of their own 'need' to supervise (Strickland, 1958; Kruglanski, 1970). Thus the role of the house co-ordinator is made more ambiguous. If specialist support, for example in the field of behaviour management, were available from a source *outside* the staffed housing service, then it could be called in by the house co-ordinator directly, avoiding demand on the centre.

However, as we noted in our comments on Table 6.2, the co-ordinators and companions shared the same view on the distribution of available support. The atmosphere in the houses was 'more intense', as one ex-nurse expressed it, and the problems that occur were more rapidly identified with the house a whole. All staff responded to management in similar ways, and as we reported in Chapter Five, found themselves in a rather more ambiguous situation than any group in the hospital. One consequence of this was an inevitable heightening of the distance between the house and the project management.

The ambiguity of role which we have recorded was also mentioned by house companions. Our data on support indicated that ambiguity was associated with a lower level of confidence about the work and suggested that all staff needed specific training in work skills.

The management of closure

Ambiguity was, in a different way, the main theme of the responses we received when discussing the hospital closure with staff. One established explanation for the distribution of power in organisations is the ability to cope with organisational uncertainty (Thompson, 1967; Hickson et al., 1971). Conversely, we may argue, employees are likely to look for a resolution of such uncertainty towards those whom they expect to have the power to resolve it. In the context of major organisational upheaval, when it is the very power balance itself that is being re-defined, staff may be expected to look to the nearest management level for a resolution.

Uncertainty over the nature of the hospital management was prevalent at the time of our research, as well as uncertainty associated with the closure itself. As we established in an earlier section of this chapter, the staff placed the blame for this general uncertainty well away from the local management, and this pattern was as true of senior nurses as it was of nursing assistants. However, in terms of most people's reactions, the important decisions are those which affect their immediate circumstances. There are two threads to this uncertainty as it affects staff, and consequently their morale, which we may call the strategic implications and the local implications.

At the strategic level, there is the problem of whether or not staff believe closure will take place. Although in the future it is probable that such a belief will be more readily formed – given the gradual increase in the number of closures – it is still a difficult thing for staff to accept. Long planning periods exacerbate this problem. In the case of Darenth Park, for example, Nancy Korman concluded that it is 'probably only physical demolition of parts of the hospital ... which will make this credible ...' (1984, p.147). Even so, to turn to the more immediate level, we would argue that it depends which parts are demolished. An acceptance of the fact of closure, at a strategic level, still permits most staff to continue their normal employment, since it is their immediate personal circumstances which bulk largest in their experience. However, to say that staff will only react when actions are taken which affect them is to tell only part of the story. People must perceive that changes affect them directly before they will take the steps which may lead to action (Jabes, 1978). In the context of the hospital it was the 'effective unit' that staff respond to which determines their morale, and that unit was undoubtedly the villa.

'People have started applying for jobs, and this in itself is very disheartening'

(In a villa about to close)

'Obviously if you work in a villa and that particular villa is not going to close within the next two years, obviously you don't tend to think about it. If it's like, say within a matter of say … the end of this month your villa will be closed – that will be very worrying to the morale of the staff. They won't know where they are going, because they are not informed until the last minute.'

(Charge nurse)

It was an increase in uncertainty at the local level, and in the daily work routine, which produced the most comments. For example, the 'closure' was seen in terms of its immediate effects on the way staff were moved. A villa that has lost a proportion of residents under the closure plan may be seen as having spare staff. Members of staff may be moved more frequently to other villas and, since the uncertainty attached to this is very unwelcome, staff morale declines even further in the villa scheduled to close.

Villas are closed as complete units in order to maximise revenue savings, as at Darenth Park (Korman and Glennerster, 1984), so there is an element of sudden death in what is seen at a higher level as a gradual decline. Staff were well aware of this:

'It's not the closure so much as the low morale – planning ahead is compromised. There is always that feeling that what you're doing is never going to come to anything – you may not see it through'.

(Charge nurse)

This last comment could be seen as containing a potentially startling remark: the actual closure is relegated to having a lesser effect than the pervasive feeling of low morale. The point is that, psychologically, the closure lacks the impact that other people's immediate responses can have, because of its relative remoteness. The implications for staff are tied very closely to the implementation of the villa closure schedule. The management of closure, seen from the prespective of staff and their reactions, is therefore primarily the mangement of uncertainty at the villa level.

The management of strategic uncertainty is important. Given that staff blame the District Health Authority in the way we have reported with respect to morale, the management of morale depends on a clear resolution of uncertainty at that level as early as possible in the closure programme. It is the commonly attributed experience of industries which need to reorganise frequently in order to meet demands from their operating environment, that morale can be maintained if staff understand the need for change and are confident in the management of that change (Peat, Marwick, 1986)

There are obvious implications for the role of health districts. Amongst the recommendations made by Korman, following her study of the closure of Darenth Park, was the proposal that districts need to become involved in the hospital during the rundown period and gear their local planning so as not to complicate the management of the hospital rundown. We can now refine that suggestion by adding that the notion of a 'hospital closure', in the context of what is essentially a *service development*, is an unneccessarily negative focus for staff. Of course staff need to be informed of the closure, but it is important for planning authorities, especially at district level, to emphasise the transition in care services rather than simply to present a closure plan of a particular institution. If staff are informed as early as possible of the rationale behind the plans, which set their hospital in a context of service change, rather than presenting it as an isolated closure, then it should prove easier to avoid the institutional myopia which can otherwise result. This could focus people's minds on the expansion of services which is actually occurring, rather than on a reduction of opportunities for employment.

Staff representation: unions and professional organisations

Finally we examine a parallel set of organisations, concerned with staff representation. The main purpose of our questions concerning staff representation was to chart any significant differences between the particular health and local authority situations which might have some more general importance. There are very few published scales concerning employees' responses to unions and staff associations. We examined a measure of union satisfaction (Glick, Mirvis and Harder, 1977) and the questionnaire produced by Uphoff and Dunnette (1956) which covered a wide range of factors. Eventually we devised two measures, shown in the two sections of question 39 in the appendix and based on some of the published items, and tested them during the pilot survey. The measures deal with Effectiveness and Legitimacy, since it seemed that apart from organisational reasons, individual responses towards unions would be due to one or other, if not both, of these factors. There was a partial confirmation of this in the data.

Staff representation was provided by four organisations; NALGO, NUPE, the RCN and CoHSE. There were no NALGO members in our hospital sample. Table 6.3 sets out the proportions within each.

Table 6.3
Relative size of membership of organisations providing staff representation in both services (per cent)

	Community	Hospital
NALGO	4.2	—
NUPE	8.3	3.6
RCN	—	12.1
CoHSE	—	69.6
Non members	83.3	10.3

There were no great variations between different types of staff within the hospital, other than the fact that only qualified staff were members of

83

the RCN, so that part-timers, night shift staff and men or women were equally likely to be members.

In the postal questionnaire we asked staff to complete our two attitude measures, regardless of whether they were members of unions or not. In fact there were no differences of any significance within the hospital on either measure. Non-members generally judged effectiveness in the same way as members, that is to say with a moderate reponse and with a very small variation in response. Legitimacy was endorsed with an even narrower variation, giving an average score well towards the 'agreement' side of the scale. Clearly non-members within the hospital were not generally or strongly anti-union. There were also no differences in perceived Effectiveness or Legitimacy between the organisations shown in Table 6.3.

One clear difference did emerge from our research. As Table 6.3 shows, only 12.5 per cent of the community staff were in a staff organisation compared with 85.3 per cent of hospital staff. We explored this difference both through the attitude measures in the postal questionnaire and in the interviews. Since we had asked non-members to complete these measures, we looked to see if a low score on perceived Effectiveness was reponsible, but there was no difference between the community and hospital on that account. There was, however, a difference on the measure of Legitimacy $(p < .01)$. Community staff scored less on this scale by an amount that is probably not due to chance $(p < .01)$. The scale is an attempt to measure the value of, need for, and legitimacy of staff organisations, and the difference suggests that the community staff were somewhat less sure of the role of unions and staff organisations.

We checked on this finding during our interviews, asking if community staff 'had any particular views' on unions, and why they were, or were not, members. On person said:

> 'I think there's a bit of a different attitude in the houses. There's not that mentality of leaving at the end of the shift. I don't think the staff are union minded.'

But this was not a typical response. It became clear when we categorised the responses from the interviews that most people had simply not got around to joining.

> 'I think I had a form about it, but, you know how it is, I never got around to filling it in.'

Two people said that they had tried to interest union representatives in recruiting staff but with little success. The picture to emerge, therefore, was one of a lack of organisation, rather than of strong feeling. Table 6.4

demonstrates this and gives our classification of replies to the interview question about unions: 'what about unions'?

Table 6.4
First responses to
neutrally worded question
about unions (per cent of
interview responses)

	Community staff	Hospital staff
Advised to join	5	33
Positive support for unions	20	8
Apathy	30	3
Lack of organisation	35	—
For protection	—	48
Opposed to unions	—	3
Don't know	10	8

The staff in the hospital explained their membership in one of two ways: either they were advised to join when they were first employed, or, they had joined anyway for 'protection'. There is little real difference here. Most of those who replied that they had joined when first employed, also said 'it's for protection.' The two main responses in the community were general apathy or a lack of local organisation, which together account for 65 per cent of replies. There were still a fifth of replies that were positive (eg 'I'm in favour of unions').

There could be several reasons for the situation. This was a new service, there were uncertainties about the most suitable organisation to join, and there may be local factors involved if a particular union was weak. The community staff were less convinced of the value of unions than the hospital employees, but their average response, on the measure we employed, was still in favour of organised representation. We can only conclude that if circumstances elsewhere repeat this pattern, there is likely to be a real gap in staff representation in community projects of this sort.

Staff in the hospital saw professional representation and protection as a necessary part of working with vulnerable people in a sensitive and demanding job. Staff in the community did not think that the need for representation had disappeared, though its urgency seemed to have diminished. It is clearly important that the various unions and staff associations should become more aware of the new situation.

7 Individual Responses to the Job

In this chapter we review the results we obtained on four different sorts of measures, all of which in one way or another can be thought of as outcomes for staff. We look at *job satisfaction* and those aspects of the job which cause it to vary. We examine *stress* in terms of its severity and the pattern of attributed causes, and also report an analysis of causes inferred from our other measures. We discuss *propensity to leave* in the context of orientation towards community employment. Finally, we report on *turnover* and the organisational factors we can identify which are associated with it.

Job satisfaction

The job satisfaction questionnaire which we employed was very similar to that being used by the Personal Social Services Research Unit, at the University of Kent, which was conducting research into the Care in the Community Initiative and evaluating the new services to clients (Hampson, Judge and Renshaw, 1984; Davis and Cherns, 1975). The set of 17 questions, each on a five point scale (1 to 5), covered a range labelled from 'very dissatisfied' to 'very satisfied'.

We shall discuss the results we obtained from these questions in several ways. Firstly, we shall examine the individual items for what they can tell us about aspects of the work that may be problematic, both within each setting and between settings. Secondly, we shall analyse the pattern of items for what that can tell us about the main characteristics of the work. Then we shall examine differences in these characteristics in the two settings and amongst the staff groups. Finally in this section we shall report on an analysis of the main correlates, or assumed causes, of these dimensions.

We turn first to our analysis of responses to individual aspects of the job. Because all the items comprise one scale, and are numerically scaled under the same range, we can assume that problems, or the lack of them, covered by any one item will show up as fairly major deviations from the average for all the items. (We define 'major' here as a value exceeding two standard deviations more or less than the mean). We can conduct a more rigorous analysis when we compare items between the two organisations but at this stage we are concerned to identify those ares where the staff in both organisations may not differ, but where both register an extreme response. The overall mean for all items was 3.5 but three items scored very differently. One was the item concerned with Relationships with Fellow Workers: in both settings it was associated with higher satisfaction. Two items were associated with noticeably lower satisfaction: income and opportunities for advancement.

All the items are shown in Table 7.1, which gives the values we obtained in the two organisations. Our analysis showed that there were no significant differences within the community service, and minimal differences between groups within the hospital, excluding senior nurses. The comparisons in Table 7.1, therefore, are between all staff in the staffed houses and all staff below nursing officer level in the hospital.

Table 7.1

Differences in job satisfaction items between community and hospital direct care staff (average scores)

	Community	Hospital*	Factor identification
1. Income	3.0	2.6	4
2. Job security	3.9	2.8*	4
3. Number of hours of work	3.7	4.1*	2
4. Flexibility of hours	3.7	3.9	2
5. Ease of travel to work	3.9	3.6	4
6. Management and supervision by your superiors	3.0	3.3	3
7. Relationships with fellow workers	4.4	4.3	2
8. Opportunities for advancement	3.0	2.8	1 and 4
9. Public respect for the sort of work you do	3.8	3.4	3
10. Your own accomplishments	3.5	3.6	1
11. Developing your skills	3.3	3.2	1
12. Having challenges to meet	3.2	3.5	1
13. The actual tasks you do	3.2	3.7*	1
14. The variety of tasks	3.1	3.5*	1
15. Opportunities to use your own initiative	3.2	3.7*	1
16. The physical work conditions	4.3	3.3*	3
17. Your work in general	3.5	3.9*	1

* Difference between hospital and community not due to chance ($p < .05$)
    Higher scores represent greater satisfaction

The first item is of major importance, of course, and we can link our discussion of satisfaction directly to its cause. We collected information on earnings with our questionnaire and most people (82 per cent) wrote in the amount of their normal gross earnings. We calculated annual levels for comparison in each group. At the time of the postal questionnaire the house companions in the community service reported average earnings which were 17.1 per cent higher than those reported by full time nursing assistants, but 9.9 per cent lower than those of SENs. The house co-ordinators reported average earnings which were 8.9 per cent higher than those of staff nurses. The community staff, therefore, saw themselves as slightly better off on average. The small difference in satisfaction shown in Table 7.1 reflects this, and is a difference which almost reaches conventional statistical significance levels ($p < .1$). However, during the period of our research, this situation changed. The 1987 nurses' pay award changed the balance slightly, although we cannot give the same level of analysis for the more recent situation. The important point, of course, is that the relative differential was well understood by staff. However, we did not assume that motivation to change the job was primarily driven by income differentials, and parts of our analysis in Chapter Three would indicate the reverse. As we shall report below other, intrinsic, elements of the job have a profound effect on response, and other extrinsic aspects may be more significant than shorter term pay differentials. This is a convenient point in our report, however, to point out the deleterious effects on joint planning that unsynchronised pay rounds can have. The NHS awards came in advance of the local authority review and have caused the differential to reverse at the time of writing. This is especially important for the registered nurse/house co-ordinator comparison because of a probable differential rate in the supply of qualified staff to the hospital; this is a point to which we will return when we discuss turnover.

Obviously these comments also apply to the item concerned with opportunities for advancement in Table 7.1. Here we do not have such a readily quantifiable explanation, but it is clear that both sets of employees are rather dissatisfied with what they presumably saw as truncated job horizons. We must emphasise, though, that the nature of the advancement to which staff were referring was likely to vary considerably. Within the hospital the relative responses of the different staff groups revealed one large anomaly. Enrolled nurses produced a score lower than that of any other group ($p < .05$). The limitations to this role, and the recent move to end enrolled nurse training, are probably responsible for the frustration that this result represents.

The closure programme may have reduced satisfaction within the hospital but, again, it threatened groups differentially. Registered nurses also scored lower than the average on this item. At that time, pay differentials would have encouraged registered nurses to join the community service, and discouraged enrolled nurses, but satisfaction with opportunities for advancement was low in the community as well. Here the explanation must centre on the available promotion prospects, rather than on the threat of future redundancy at the hospital. Whilst enrolled nurses were probably responding to the already reduced opportunities in the hospital, regardless of the closure, in the community all staff were aware that few opportunities existed above co-ordinator level. During the period of the research, intermediate posts were introduced but, inevitably, there were more staff hoping for such appointments than there were available positions within the new service. As we reported in Chapter Three, the community service was staffed with people who were generally looking for advancement in their careers, so these findings underline the need to ensure that the staff who are appointed vary sufficiently in their aspirations to provide a degree of stability within the organisation.

There were significant differences between the hospital and the community for six items in Table 7.1. Firstly, and for obvious reasons, satisfaction with job security was considerably lower in the hospital. The closure programme had approximately eight years to run at the time the study took place, so that in reality many people had considerable job security. However, uncertainty about the progress of the plan was demoralising for all staff and this emphasises the need for information about the plan to be communicated as soon as possible.

Community staff expressed dissatisfaction with their hours of work, as Table 7.1 shows. There were two aspects to this difference. Firstly, all the community staff reported working extra hours. The reasons for this varied but the closeness of the relationships between staff and residents accounted for a degree of out-of-hours contact. Mainly, however, the extra time was to cover for shortage of staff or to allow for more convenient or extended overlaps of duty. Secondly, this lower satisfaction almost certainly related to the pattern of hours. The shift system in the community service tended to concentrate staff hours into long bouts. As we shall see later in the chapter, this aspect of the work was also associated with stress.

Table 7.1 presents two items relating directly to the nature of the work: these were 'the actual tasks you do' and 'the variety of tasks'. As we reported in Chapter Five, the community staff described the two task dimensions of their job in a way which did not differ in any noticeable manner from the average in the hospital. Now, however, we can see that they were much less satisfied with these two items than were their opposite numbers working in the hospital. The range of 'actual tasks' you do and the 'variety' of tasks provided rather less satisfaction for staff in the community, even though their jobs were seen to be about as varied as jobs in the hospital. Clearly we have now encountered differences that are more likely to be due to variations between sorts of people rather than sorts of circumstances. We will examine this issue in the next paragraph but first we will record the final item which reveals a major difference. 'The physical work conditions' in the ordinary house environment were regarded more favourably than the average hospital conditions. This is perhaps an unsurprising result but, as we shall see, relates to more than just the comfort of a homely setting.

Any job satisfaction measure may vary according to the people who respond and according to the circumstances to which they respond. The community staff, for example, were different in a number of ways from the average hospital employee, as we have recorded, so that the differences in satisfaction scores may also reflect differences in them as people. Their motivations and expectations were different, so we can assume that their reported level of satisfaction varied to some extent because of this rather than because of actual differences in the circumstances.

It is of course problematic to establish such differences by looking solely at individual items from the questionnaire; we miss the additional information contained in those items which are less noticeably different, but which together may add up to a significant pattern. Our next analysis therefore combined all the items according to the way in which people responded to them. We used a technique called Principal Component Analysis for this task. This technique examines the way people respond to each item in terms of how they respond to all the others. In other words it asks whether being more satisfied on a particular item usually means being less satisfied on another or more satisfied on a third and so on. The outcome of this analysis is a set of separate factors each of which combines a number of items. Again, the exact values produced are numerically arbitrary but the pattern that emerges is valuable if it has validity; that is, if it confirms what has been found by other research. The results we obtained reflect what is known in the literature about the main dimensions of job satisfaction, The final column of Table 7.1 shows the pattern that emerged. We found four factors, which combine the items in the way shown. We have chosen the following labels for these factors:

1   Self-development
2   Convenience and Friendship
3   Status
4   Extrinsic Rewards

The labels we have chosen represent our descriptions of what we think underlies the responses to the items linked by this sort of analysis. For example, the items which have the greatest effect on Factor 1 are related to intrinsic rewards associated with personal growth. Note that the 'task' items fall into this factor and this is undoubtedly due to the fact that they reflect frustration which has its origins in the staff, as we suggested above.

Factor 2, which we called 'Convenience and Friendship', concerns the way in which the job 'fits in' with people's requirements. This factor includes the number of hours of work, the convenience of those hours and relationships with fellow workers. Given the very high proportion of women in the occupation, this factor probably reflects the kind of judgements people make in job choice. The hospital represents a convenient job to many people in the local neighbourhood, providing part-time or full-time work alongside other staff who may often be neighbours or friends, or, indeed spouses.

Factor 3, which we called 'Status', is rather different. It represents judgements about the nature of the work and its conditions, combining public respect and working conditions. We did not set out to measure status in the postal questionnaire so it is interesting to see it appear in a way which accords with our findings at interview. One concern over community care involves public reactions to the residents, so we asked about the responses people had experienced when first they came to work with mentally handicapped people. This was a question to which almost everyone could respond.

A simple categorisation of the remarks that people reported showed that a majority had encountered positive, approving judgements (43.1 per cent) but many had encountered mixed or predominantly negative reactions (29.4 per cent). There was no clear difference between settings but, of course, the community service was fairly new, so many staff were reporting reactions to their *first* employment with people with mental handicap. Often comments centred on the hospital rather than on the residents, in a way which reflected the stigma which can attach to such institutions or to the people in them (Goffman, 1964; Jones and Fowles,

1984). Characterisation of the work by the public can reflect, therefore, on the nature and conditions of work (Saunders, 1981).

Factor 4 concerns the 'extrinsic' rewards of the work: it brings together income, job security and travel costs and 'opportunities for advancement'. The latter has implications for income as well as for self-development and thus also appears partially in Factor 1.

Having outlined this procedure and some of its results, we can now review the differences revealed between the community and hospital. We will concentrate on Factor 1, but will first briefly discuss the other three factors which, together, have much less effect than the first factor alone. Our item analysis of Factor 4 showed that the community staff were more satisfied with the level of their Extrinsic Rewards. However, we have already noted that this finding is likely to vary as the wage rates change. Analysis of Factor 2, convenience and friendship, showed no differences between the two sets of staff. Factor 3, which was concerned with status, showed that the community staff were more satisfied with this aspect of the work than most groups of staff in the hospital. We can only speculate on the reasons for this. It is possible that the real difference in physical work conditions is associated with a different public response to staff who work in the community. However, it could be simply that the response reflects staff optimism about the success of the community initiative.

We turn now to Factor 1. Whereas community staff were relatively more satisfied with status and extrinsic rewards, they were rather less satisfied with self development aspects. Given what we have reported concerning staff motivation and beliefs, it seems very likely that this difference was due to the staff in the community service being generally more highly motivated and more ambitious, with relatively higher expectations than the hospital staff. Furthermore, these aspects of the work were probably influential in the choice of career, and, in the choice of a community based service. Despite the slight monetary advantage at the time, as one house companion put it:

> 'It's not that you don't need the money, but that's not why you do it, is it.'

In common with other research concerned with nurses (Benton and White, 1972; Nnadozie and Eldar, 1985), we found that accounts of job satisfaction were dominated by the intrinsic aspects of the work. In our interviews we found that just over half of the staff in both settings spontaneously mentioned resident-centred aspects such as teaching objectives, witnessing change or just being with the residents. Only a minority spoke of extrinsic factors first (10 per cent and 17 per cent in community and hospital respectively). The items in Factor 1, however, are at a slightly higher level of abstraction and are concerned with more general sources of reward and personal growth. We have already referred to sources of instability in the community service, to the age range and life-cycle stages of the staff, now we add that the lower level of satisfaction with the potential of the service to meet self development aspects suggests a further source of dissatisfaction. Another distinction needs to be made at this point, however. In our discussion of item 8 in Table 7.1, 'opportunities for advancement', we concentrated on an interpretation of this as it reflected *career* development. In fact this item divides between Factors 1 and 4. Although it mostly contributes to *self-development*, it also contributes to extrinsic rewards. Thus Factor 1 is to some extent about 'getting on' and not just about intrinsic rewards. The lack of a difference on item 8 is thus partially resolved by this finding, which suggests that rather more professional ambition is present among community staff.

What contributes to this relative lack of satisfaction with the self-development aspects of the job in the community? Our research was partly designed to answer this question. We have reported variations in a number of measures of different aspects of the work: the basic dimensions of the work, aspects of the work role, the nature of the organisation as it is seen by staff and the level of support from immediate superiors. Thus we can determine which of these aspects are responsible for producing the variation in satisfaction with self-development which we have recorded. We applied a regression analysis to achieve this. Regression analysis calculates how much effect each of the set of possible causes has on the outcome measure, whilst simultaneously allowing for any effects which those 'causes' may have on one another. Given the 'arbitrary' values of the outcome measure we note that such a casual analysis would normally present some technical problems of interpretation, but our requirements were rather more descriptive, and our main concern was with the comparison of two different settings. Thus we applied the technique separately to the community staff and to hospital staff up to the level of charge nurse/sister. The results are summarised in Table 7.2.

Table 7.2
Aspects of the job which significantly affect satisfaction with self-development amongst community and hospital staff

Predictors	Index of effect (betas)	
	Community	Hospital
Task variety	.49	—
Role Ambiguity	− .42	− .35
Feedback	—	.22

(The size of the effects is not due to chance p $<$ .001)

Table 7.2 shows that two aspects of the job in the community appeared to have an effect which was greater than might be expected by chance. The index reported in Table 7.2 shows both the relative strength of each aspect and gives the direction of the effect and can vary from minus one to plus one. In other words the positive value for task variety shows that satisfaction with self-development was greater when variety was greater, whilst the negative value for Role Ambiguity shows that satisfaction was reduced by greater ambiguity.

Here we encounter a major problem in the operation of the community service. In order to produce and maintain a quality service, staff are chosen for their beliefs and commitment. These staff are mostly young and ambitious, they have high expectations and high needs for self development. They are doing a job which offers a level of variety similar to that reported in the hospital but appear to seek additional variety to satisfy their need to develop their skills. At the same time they are noticeably unsure of their exact role. This combination of relative confusion and lack of challenge is a powerful endorsement of the specific training requirements which staff reported to us, and which we discuss in Chapter Eight.

However, whilst training is undoubtedly required, changing the job is only one solution, or part of a solution, to the problems apparent here. A change in the typical composition of the work force is another possibility. There is a conundrum here. If staff with somewhat lower aspirations for self development are employed, will this simply lower motivation and produce poorer performance? If staff with higher development needs continue to dominate the service, will they become bored and frustrated and quickly move on? Both tendencies seem likely to continue, and a balanced staff is needed in order to temper the worst of both effects, aided by appropriately focused training and supervision.

In the hospital we see that the much wider range of aspirations and needs produces a different answer to the question 'what causes lower satisfaction with self development? In the more stable and established environment of the hospital, it is not primarily a lack of variety that accounts for variation in satisfaction. Role Ambiguity has the greater effect, combined with performance Feedback. Again, the signs of the index indicate that more ambiguity reduced satisfaction whilst more feedback increased it. Personal development, skill growth and accomplishment are less limited by variation in the tasks but more by some confusion over the appropriate role and effectiveness of action. Uncertainty in the matter of the work itself is a hallmark of professional occupations (Elliott, 1972) so that some level of ambiguity in the role, representing the interaction of professional training and implementation, is to be expected. The contrast with the community service is mainly one of scale; expecting a more demanding role, but being relatively unprepared by specialist training, left the community staff rather more dissatisfied with the range of the job and uncertain as to how they should fit into it. This would seem a very likely pattern in a new service and reinforces our belief that as full a management structure as possible should be set up at the start of such a service, backed by adequate induction training.

Dissatisfaction and stress There is, as yet, no agreed model for the ways in which various job factors relate to the production of stress at work. The contribution of stress to job performance, temporary withdrawal and quitting is not clear (Jamal, 1984). However, as we explained in our chapter on methods, many of the most important factors implicated in the generation of stress have been documented (Cooper and Payne, 1978) and found to predict dissatisfaction amongst nurses (Gray-Toft and Anderson, 1981; Cartwright, 1979). Our main concerns were to detect any significant variations in stress between organisations and groups, to relate the levels of stress to other work factors and to identify specific stresses which also might be characteristic of the organisation.

Stress has been linked to job satisfaction (Lyons, 1971; Miles, 1975) but it is more likely to be those factors which relate to intrinsic satisfaction that are implicated. Herzberg originally proposed that intrinsic factors produce satisfaction, whilst extrinsic factors produce dissatisfaction. As we reported above, the overall level of satisfaction with extrinsic factors was low in both organisations. However, stress has been linked to satisfaction via role ambiguity, and this has been linked to supervisory style (Gray-Toft and Anderson, 1985). So we would expect the sort of results we obtained and summarized in table 5.2. Whatever the nature of the relationship, the level of stress generated is of interest, and may be critical (Ivancevich and Matteson, 1981). Thus we decided to measure stress and chose to do this with the Malaise Inventory (Rutter et al., 1970a, 1970b, 1975).

The Malaise Inventory consists of 24 questions about physical and emotional health, scored zero or one for 'no' and 'yes' answers respectively, and summed to produce an overall score. We chose this particular measure because it is well validated (Bebbington and Quine, 1986), has been used in studies of carers of handicapped children (Bradshaw et al., 1982) and by two of the present authors in a study of parents caring for children with a mental handicap (Pahl and Quine, 1985). Thus we anticipated that comparisons could be made between staff employed in the two service settings and parent carers.

The results we obtained are shown in Table 7.3 which includes, for comparison, the results of the other studies mentioned above.

Table 7.3
Mean malaise scores

Study	Score
Pahl and Quine (1985) Parents of mentally handicapped children	5.8
Bradshaw et al. (1982) Parents of ESN(S) children	5.7
Rutter (1970) Parents of normal children	3.2
The present study: Community staff	3.04
Hospital staff	2.74

Table 7.3 shows that those who are employed to work in the mental handicap services have significantly lower stress scores than mothers caring at home for children with mental handicaps. The differences between the stress scores of those employed in the hospital and in the community service

were not statistically significant. We therefore concluded that the stress levels in the job do not vary in any important way between the organisations. However, an acceptable level in one setting may be problematic in another. We must ask, therefore, about the causes of stress and examine the circumstances associated with it to ensure that there are no critical differences hidden within this average.

Firstly, we can extend the analysis of the Malaise Inventory to include those factors which may exert a systematic effect on it, in the way in which we examined job satisfaction. We conducted regression analyses using the set of variables to which we have so far referred, including the two measures of resident characteristics. In the parallel study of parent carers it was the presence of disturbed behaviour which had the greatest effect on stress (Quine, 1986). Factors such as the isolation of the carer also contributed to higher stress levels. Thus we could anticipate that those variables that refer to supervision and interpersonal contact might moderate the levels of stress experienced by staff working with a higher proportion of behaviourally disturbed residents.

In fact the results do not show any such effects, rather they reinforce the findings discussed at the beginning of this section in that it is role factors and the related organisational aspects which account for the significant part of the variation in the Malaise score. Table 7.4 summarizes the results from two separate analyses.

Table 7.4
Significant predictors of stress in community and hospital staff

Predictors	Index of effect (betas)	
	Community	Hospital
Role Ambiguity	.71	—
Autonomy	.51	—
Role Conflict	—	.23
Resident Interaction	—	− .14

(The size of the effects is not due to chance $p < .001$)

Table 7.4 shows that community staff were more likely to have higher stress scores if they were experiencing high levels of Role Ambiguity, combined with high levels of Autonomy, in their jobs. When we recall that our measure of Autonomy reflects being left alone to act without supervision, we can see that it was coping alone with a relatively ill defined role that contributed most to stress in the staffed houses.

In the hospital, the pattern was different, even though the level of stress was similar. Staff were more likely to be stressed when their jobs involved high levels of Role Conflict, that is to say when there was a conflict between the way in which they wanted to carry out their role and the way in which they were able to do so. The negative sign attached to the effect of Resident Interaction shows that it is *reductions* in individual resident contact that are associated with increased stress. Thus we have a picture of staff trying to do a job which they conceive of in one way but are obliged by the circumstances in the hospital to do in another and which, we may surmise, involves them in resource problems which are reflected in their lack of contact with individual residents.

These are, as we stated, overall analyses. We could not examine separate villas or houses adequately with these measures. However, the results presented in Table 7.4 are from analyses which initially included measures of resident characteristics. Those measures exerted little or no effect on stress. Amongst parent carers it was the management of difficult behaviour which increased stress. In the hospital stress appeared to be the result of having to care for large numbers of people in a manner which limited individual contact.

We followed up the possible causes of stress at interview. We cannot directly link our questionnaire and interview measurements, but we can characterise the pattern of attributed causes in the two settings. They are somewhat different. Table 7.5 lists the categories of responses to questions about stress at work for the two organisations. The proportions given refer to first and second comments combined.

Table 7.5

Attributed causes of stress (per cent of interview responses)

	Community	Hospital
No real problems	47.1	55.0
Sleeplessness	14.7	—
Management/pressure from above	14.7	5.0
Behaviour problems	—	12.5
Staff shortage	5.9	8.8
Work overload	8.8	5.0
Intensity of involvement	8.8	—
Uncertainty	—	5.0
Other	—	8.8

We have not conducted a rigorous statistical analysis of the proportions in this table because it would be inappropriate. For example, the community staff did not cite behaviour problems directly as a cause of stress, but it is behavioural disturbance at night that contributes to the category of sleeplessness. This latter category relates directly to the shift system to which we referred in Chapter Five. Unlike the Nimrod staffed housing project, which employs part-time night staff, the present service sought to provide continuity of care by the same persons (Evans et al., 1984). Thus the 'sleep-in' shift, with its special allowance, was adopted. The problem is that this 'shift' is assumed to involve minimal activity, and no doubt does in many cases. Where there is disruption, however, or where, for example, individual staff find sleeping-in difficult, the broken night can result in staff stress on the following day.

Similarly it was difficult to separate replies about staff shortage from the category 'work overload'. Because of the minimal staffing levels, such shortage, usually occasioned by absence, was a problem in both settings. Together these two categories probably do refer to overload, and account for very similar proportions in both settings. Intensity of involvement, however, refers solely to the atmosphere in the staffed houses. As some hospital staff explained, the stress induced on a villa could be coped with because it could be 'isolated' from the rest of the person's life.

> 'You're only here for your shift and I live so far away from the place, I've got no contact with the problems. I can get away from it.'
>
> (Charge nurse)

But the community staff seemed to work at a more intense level.

> 'I find it difficult to shut down at the end of the day. If a situation arises (within the house) and it isn't resolved by the end of the day, then I find it very, very difficult to switch off.'
>
> (House companion)

Whilst such variations are obviously personal in nature, some staff did attribute a pervasive sense of intensity to the service as a whole, and this may have reflected the type of people selected for the job. However, we did not find a significant difference between the overall stress levels, as we reported above, so if such tendencies existed, we did not record them. It is possible that loyalty to the organisation, as reflected in our findings on morale, and commitment to the ideal of community service, as revealed in our analysis of beliefs, acts to moderate or compensate for the stressful nature of the work pattern by motivating performance in the face of stress, rather than creating withdrawal from it. There is some general occupational evidence that such effects can occur (Bartol, 1979; Greenhaus, 1971; Weiner and Vardi, 1980) and partial support for it amongst nurses (Jamal, 1984).

In summary, it is being left to confront the ambiguity of a new professional role that contributes most to stress in the community, but being obliged by circumstances to work differently from the preferred way that contributes most to stress in the hospital. One house companion, who had previously worked as a nurse in the hospital, described the sources of stress in the two settings in a way which expressed in personal terms the more general findings coming from our analysis.

> '[speaking about the house] When you're on duty, you're there right – can't relax because you're there all the time. You need to be aware what's going on all the time – you have to keep your eye on them. If [a resident] wants to do something, then I've got to supervise, so the others have to sit around.
> [Compared to hospital?] More. More (stress) in this job than in the hospital. The targets (in the hospital) are impossible. On some wards maybe it's different, but on the one I was on, no. In the [community service] they are achievable but you've really got to work to it. [So in the hospital it's frustration?] Yes, you can't win.'

Again, however, we must emphasise that our analysis of stress was at a general level. The job could and did vary considerably between villas in the hospital, and between houses in the community service. In the hospital the different villas tended to house different sorts of people so the concentration of particular sorts of residents was common: elderly women, disturbed men and so on (cf. Alaszewski, 1986). In the community there was no comparable 'specialisation', so people with individual problems tended to define the characteristic pattern within each house. In the hospital there was a reserve of expertise available but, in both organisations, the response to stress-inducing situations tended to be crisis management. This reflected the resource levels, of course, especially staffing, but organisational flexibility also varied. Staffing levels within the hospital tended to reflect the dependency level of a given villa, or the redefined task structure in a half-way house, but shift arrangements were stable. In the community the organisational structure and shifts were also fixed, but for reasons of scale there was not much reserve capacity for routine cover and very little spare expert help. Being able to call on a reserve of staff would assist in the more extreme cases of disturbance, but where the pattern of behaviour in a given house is very different from others it could be that some organisational flexibility would help to reduce stress. For example, if one resident habitually disturbs the sleep of the others, including the 'sleep-in' staff member, the pattern of day-sleep-in-day shifts is more stressful and less efficient than in other houses where night disruptions are rare. In such cases different shift arrangements might alleviate the problem.

Thinking about leaving and thinking about community work

All employers must be concerned about the loss of staff: in the health service this issue is particularly acute, since staff costs are the largest single item in a health authority's budget. Major re-structuring, of the sort currently occurring in the mental handicap services, involves the additional question of whether staff will be willing to adapt to the new patterns of employment. Two sections of the questionnaire were concerned with the staffs' intentions with regard to future employment, we have described these as Propensity to Leave and Orientation towards Community Employment.

At the beginning of the research, it was not clear what information we could obtain about 'leavers' and, of course, it was uncertain how many staff would leave within the timespan of the research. We decided to include a measure of 'Propensity to Leave', since such measures have been reported to be highly correlated with actual turnover (Miller, Katerborg and Hulin, 1979). We drew items from the work of Lyons (1971) and Seashore et al. (1982) to produce a measure scaled from 2 to 10. It combined likelihood of leaving with the contemplation of leaving. Similarly we thought to measure how people were responding to the notion of community employment. We developed a two item scale (scored 2 to 8) which combined likelihood of seeking such employment, 'if for some reason you were to lose your job here', with the degree of concern shown if such a post were to be unavailable. We assumed therefore that we would be measuring commitment to such employment in the community.

What did we find? Firstly, a simple comparison between the direct care staff of the hospital and the community staff showed scores of 5.75 and

6.5 on Propensity to Leave. The difference suggested that community staff were more likely to leave than hospital staff. The difference turned out to be a chance variation, according to statistical tests. However, as we showed in Chapter Two, the community scheme *did* have a greater turnover rate during the period of the study. So we have some justification for assuming that our measure was showing a real difference. This is important because the rationale for a decision to leave is often obscure, and thinking about leaving is neither the same as actually leaving nor does it necessarily have the same meaning for different people (Steers and Mowday, 1980). Our use of a confidential serial number on the questionnaires permitted us to identify those staff who left employment during the following 18 months. Subsequently we could add this fact to our data file and analyse the characteristics of those who had left to compare them with those who had stayed.

We will discuss some of those characteristics, as they relate to various aspects of the hospital organisation, in the final section of this chapter. Here, however, we will note two things which argue for the efficiency of our measure of Propensity to Leave and which, consequently, permitted us to make useful comparisons between the two organisations. The community service did not lose a large enough number of staff for us to examine in any detail the connections between the decision to leave and organisational factors. If our measure of Propensity to Leave was a good predictor of *actual* leaving, however, we could analyse variations in that measure using the whole sample. We have already referred to one aspect, namely that the measure showed a slightly higher Propensity to Leave in the community and this was confirmed by actual turnover. Since we could identify subsequent leavers, however, we could also test to see if the measure was significantly higher amongst people who *had* left both organisations. In fact it was considerably higher. Those who had left the hospital scored 7.1 on average, compared with 5.3 for those who were still employed 18 months after the measures were taken. This is a very large difference, unlikely to be due to chance ($p < .0001$). Those who left the community scheme scored 6.9 compared with 5.6 for those who stayed. This is a similar kind of difference, although because of the small number of leavers (8), statistical tests record a probability higher than that conventionally accepted ($p < .09$). These differences tend to confirm the predictive capacity of the Propensity to Leave measure. So we examined the factors which led to increases in that propensity in both settings. Table 7.6 shows the results of multiple regression analyses using the job, role, organisational, satisfaction, stress and support variables together with age, length of service, beliefs and resident characteristics to predict Propensity to Leave. Again only those factors which produced an effect are listed.

The table shows that, in the community, it is the factors of Role Ambiguity and Autonomy which are linked to higher scores for Propensity to Leave. We have recorded previously that stress was associated with being left to confront the ambiguity of a new role. Now we can add that the same process leads to people having more thoughts about leaving.

Table 7.6

Factors affecting
propensity to leave in
community and hospital

| | Index of effect (betas) | |
	Community	Hospital
Role Ambiguity	.80	.12
Autonomy	.42	—
Interpersonal Interaction	—	.23
Service Orientation	—	.17
Age	(− .3 at p < .08)	− .32
	—	− .23
Satisfaction (self development)	—	− .18
Satisfaction (status)	—	− .16
Community Employment Orientation	—	− .15
Satisfaction (extrinsic rewards)		

(The size of the effects is not due to chance p < .01)

In the hospital there was a somewhat different reaction. Table 7.6 shows that Role Ambiguity did have some effect, but not in conjunction with the relative isolation represented by our Measure of Autonomy. Rather it was people who engaged in more interpersonal interaction who had the higher Propensity to Leave. But the single biggest effect was that due to age. The negative sign shows that it was younger staff who expressed the greater Propensity to Leave, and that those thinking about leaving were less satisfied with the rewards offered by the job. Those thinking most about leaving also tended to be in favour of the community type of service but were less likely to be thinking of seeking employment in such service.

Summarizing these results suggests that those who were considering leaving the hospital were active younger staff, seeking opportunities for self-development and higher status and money; although they tended to support the community service idea, they were not, themselves, particularly oriented towards work in the community. Leaving the hospital is about being young and ambitious; leaving the community is about being unsure of the job and the responsibility. It is interesting that age also features in the explanation for community responses, but just fails to meet the statistical criterion (of p < .05). But in any setting, it is the young who can afford to leave (March and Simon, 1958) and this is certainly true in, for example, social work generally (Knapp et al., 1981) as well as in long-term care institutions (George, 1983). Of course most of the employees in the community service *were* young, so their potential mobility was higher than that of staff in the hospital.

What is also interesting is that the Community Employment Orientation did not differ between the two organisations. On our measure, the community staff scored an average of 5.33, the hospital staff a value of 5.57. This is not a statistically significant difference. So although the community staff were highly committed to the *idea* of a community service, they did not think it any more likely than did hospital staff that they would work again in such a service. Indeed, as we have just seen, those with a higher Propensity to Leave the hospital were even less likely to be thinking about community jobs. This is, in other words, a picture of potential wastage to the service as a whole, where by 'wastage' we mean the permanent loss of people from the particular labour market, rather than from any one organisation served by it.

In the interviews we asked several questions concerning employment intentions, in an attempt to estimate potential wastage and organisational stability. In addition we collected information on the destinations of those who actually left the community service during the period. There were no comparable data for the hospital. Of those who left the community service, exactly half went to jobs involving care for people with mental handicaps, and most of the rest to other community type jobs, which confirms a considerable level of wastage to the community services as a whole. With the small numbers involved we could not, and did not intend, to produce a detailed survey of actual turnover. There are useful reviews on the subject of turnover (Pettman, 1973; Price, 1977) including in the field of nursing (Mercer, 1979). Rather our focus was on the possible differences between settings, and the potential for movement between them.

We asked about immediate and longer term intentions in both settings. Table 7.7 summarizes the responses to the first of these questions. We have shown 'improvement to career' as a separate category. It represents a 'change' from current employment, since such improvements were typically defined in terms of leaving the hospital or the community service houses. In the latter case, however, we included the hope of promotion within the social services department.

Table 7.7
Immediate future employment intentions (per cent of interview responses)

	Community	Hospital
Improvement to career	47.1	12.2
All other kinds of move, including giving up work	11.8	19.5
Remaining in present job	29.4	63.4
Uncertain	11.8	6.9

The pattern within the hospital was not dependent on staff grade. The Propensity to Leave measure did record a significant linear trend ($p < .05$) with a sharp, but not statistically significant, jump in propensity between enrolled nurses and registered nurses, but actual turnover proportions were the same, as we showed in Chapter Two. In Table 7.7 therefore, the grades are grouped together in the hospital column.

Thus there are strong indications that job characteristics are reflected in Propensity to Leave within the community, and a reflection of this in the hospital sample. But strategic thinking is likely to be different in form from the often reactive decision involved in leaving at a particular time. People may join an organisation intending to leave and may subsequently leave, or indeed, may subsequently stay as the result of changes in circumstances

(Mercer, 1979). We tried, therefore, to get at the strategic thinking of the staff. What we reported about the youth and ambition of the community staff was demonstrated again in these replies. Nearly half had some sort of approximate plan for the next few years, usually involving movement out of the direct care role. There is clearly a potential instability here and, although the translation of intention into action is not straightforward, the comparison with the hospital is nevertheless quite clear. The strategies of the more youthful community staff tended to be less defined than those of hospital staff, reflecting both the different organisational structures and also a more fluid response to occupational opportunity. Ambition in the hospital tended to reflect knowledge of the career structure, while in the community it revealed an acceptance of a wide range of possibilities in the general area of care for mentally handicapped people. The other element in the hospital concerned awareness of community employment options. This was poorly developed since, as Table 7.7 shows, most people were not intending to move in the immediate future. Replies tended to be general. We prompted people to consider what they would do if their intentions were thwarted by circumstances in the hospital and in reply 17.5 per cent mentioned some form of community work. The simplest, and of course, immediately least costly choice is well represented by this exchange:

> [Immediate intentions?] 'I would like to stay in mental handicap nursing, either to work in the community or a group home. I intend to do my years out with the mentally handicapped.'
> [When might you think of leaving?] 'Oh I'll stay here until the hospital closes.'

We re-analysed these responses to get some sort of estimate of possible wastage. Table 7.8 summarizes our categorisation of replies according to whether staff anticipated working with the same client group. Of course a large proportion in the hospital intended to 'stay with the sinking ship', as one put it, and this inflates the number in that category, but the comparison highlights the more fluid response in the new service.

Table 7.8
Proportion of staff intending to remain with client group (per cent of interview responses)

	Community	Hospital
Remain with client group	41.2	63.4
Not necessarily stay with client group	35.3	29.3
Uncertain	23.5	7.3

The main thing to emerge from these various analyses is the comparison between the two settings. If we count staff who were uncertain in their intentions as being likely to stay in their present position, then one way to represent this comparison is in terms of the proportions of staff intending to remain with the client group. In the case of immediate intentions, these proportions are 41 per cent in the community and 63 per cent in the hospital. In the case of longer term intentions, these figures change to 29 per cent in the community and 54 per cent in the hospital.

This picture reflects the levels of actual turnover, reported in Chapter Two. As Mercer notes in his examination of the prediction of turnover, the greatest effect is due to 'the nurses' own expression of their future work intention'. (Mercer, 1979).

Looking forward, by examining intentions, seems a legitimate and valuable exercise on this evidence. Surprisingly, perhaps, the established but closing institution has greater staff stability into the near future than the developing community service. As closure approaches and the community service matures, this balance will almost certainly change. From the responses it seemed likely that a large part of the hospital workforce, who by now certainly believe in the closure, were intending to sit it out. Recruitment, then, will become crucial if the usual rate of leaving is maintained.

In the community it is retention that appears to be the greater problem. What organisational lessons can we learn about successful retention in the longer established environment of the hospital? The two relevant factors seem to be shift patterns and hours worked. Both of these are different between the two settings. In Table 7.9 we show the average length of service of different groups of hospital staff: those who worked part time, or on the night shift, were likely to have given more years of service to the hospital than full time staff on the day shift.

Table 7.9
Average length of service (years) for different shifts and time worked

Overall	(N = 202)	7.69 years		
All day shift	6.80 (143)		All night shift	10.00 (59)
Full time	6.03 (126)		Full time	11.10 (24)
Part time	12.20 (17)		Part time	9.20 (35)

Thus, in the hospital, both shift arrangements and the possibility of part-time working contributed substantially to the stability of the workforce. An analysis of variance confirms that these differences are not chance effects ($p < .05$). As we reported in Chapter Three the varied work patterns that were available made the job convenient for many staff and especially for married women. As the domestic circumstances of staff change, they can usually arrange for a related change in their hours or shift. This suggests that the employment of part-time staff would add to the stability of the community service. Of course the night shift in the hospital carries an additional salary allowance, but it may be that a combination of different arrangements could be made to suit the individual character of the houses. An alternative would be the provision of a more flexible pool of part-time staff. However, in the hospital such flexibility was not without problems. Being moved at short notice was mentioned by all those who had experienced it as something which they did not particularly like, which 'prevented teamwork', made them feel exploited and so on. This was probably just a reaction to a new working situation but it could be that too much flexibility would reduce the attractiveness of the job. Certainly the hospital should be aware that its part-time employees are a valuable resource, adding great stability at a time of run-down.

Two more factors need to be included as contributions to stability. We have already reported on the characteristics of the workforce in both organisations and we noted the differences in the distributions of ages and genders. Clearly younger people are more mobile and the concentration of a youthful staff in a community service will add to instability. The presence of male staff, however, is also important. One aim of the community project was to balance gender in its service and there is some reason to believe that this was an achievable goal, given that at the qualified level the proportion of male staff in the hospital was 42 per cent (close to the national proportion of 43 per cent male RNMH). But there is a more complicated relationship here between reasons for working and pattern of employment.

In view of the recent attention paid to discrimination in the NHS (Davies and Rosser, 1986; Dingwall, 1972), we asked about the differences in promotion and job prospects between men and women. In the community 86 per cent of the staff agreed that there was no difference, and should be none. In the hospital the comparable figure was 71 per cent, while 21 per cent thought that men should get more promotion. Whatever staff may have thought about it, however, the proportions of men in the different staff grades increased throughout the hierarchy. Table 7.10 shows that very few men were unqualified nursing assistants.

Table 7.10
Proportions of men at each grade (per cent)

Director and senior nurses	67
Charge nurses and sisters	64
Staff nurses	30
SENs	28
Nursing assistants	14

This tallies with what would be expected from the career orientation and movement of men in nursing as a whole (Dingwall and McIntosh, 1978). But it raises the question of career progression for all staff and the relative opportunities in the community. The longer average length of full time service of men was reflected in their tenure of more senior positions. There were only two men in our questionnaire survey who were working part-time. Amongst full-time staff below senior level, men had on average 9.7 years of service compared with 5.1 years for women. Whatever the complexities of motivation and differential selection which may have been operating here, however, the stability represented by these figures is true only within certain of the grades. Figure 7.1 shows the average length of service for the grades by men and women.

Statistical tests showed that the retention of staff over time increased linearly with seniority for women (p < .02) but not for men. Instead in the case of men, there were deviations at particular grades, most obviously at the enrolled nurse grade, which here included senior enrolled nurses. The

Figure 7.1

The average length of service of men and women in different staff grades

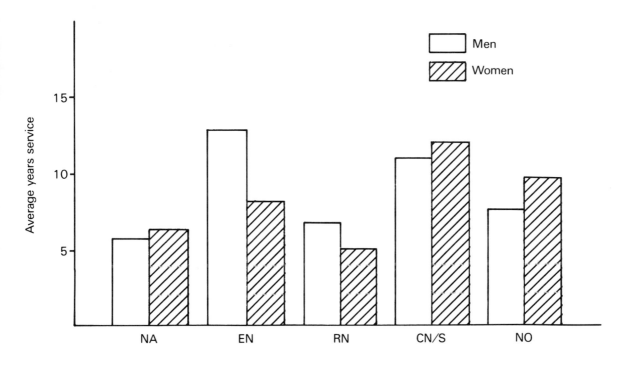

greater stability of this grade has been established before (Mercer, 1979, p.50). The decrease in the average length of service at higher grades, combined with the higher proportions of men in these grades, can only be interpreted in terms of mobility in and out of the hospital. Women who have progressed through this hierarchy have tended to remain in the same institution. We can confirm this interpretation quite simply by comparing the total length of service of male and female staff in mental handicap care. This comparison shows that the senior men have much longer overall service than appears in Figure 7.1 and indicates the importance of mobility.

We must take into account the differential propensity to move out of the local labour market that is indicated here. Now that community jobs are beginning to appear, and opportunities within the hospital are declining, those seeking to advance must more readily contemplate moving. We have seen that younger staff are doing this, but the tendency for men to move out of the area to other hospitals more freely than women may continue, assuming that the cultural factors underlying it persist into the near future. Since there are community jobs at a similar level of pay, but with possibly reduced career opportunities, these may attract more female hospital staff than male staff as closure approaches. Certainly the most common first job move would be to the charge nurse/sister grade, where numbers of posts have been reduced by the closure. As Figure 7.1 shows (and statistical tests confirm) there is no substantial difference in the length of service of registered nurses and nursing assistants. This suggests that female registered nurses would be more likely to take up community posts, if we assume that the nursing assistants are less geographically mobile and that when *they* leave it will be, as we discussed above, only because the hospital is closing. Certainly with the small proportion of men in the nursing assistant grade, it is difficult to see how the proportion of men in a community service can be maintained from a hospital supply, even if the pay differential at registered nurse level is minimised.

We attempted to illuminate the issue of labour mobility by questions in the interview about geographical mobility and about the status of earnings. Table 7.11 shows a categorisation of answers to the first of these questions.

Table 7.11
Geographical mobility of community staff, qualified and unqualified hospital staff (per cent of interview responses)

Willing to move	Community staff	Qualified (hospital)	Unqualified (hospital)
Within local area only	29.4	47.4	81.8
Elsewhere	70.6	52.6	18.2

(The differences are not due to chance $p < .01$)

Further checks showed that qualified staff were significantly more willing to move than the unqualified, as would be expected, and that the community staff had an even higher willingness to move.

During the period of our research the nurses' pay settlement altered the balance which had existed in favour of the community posts. There had been a differential which provided an incentive for nursing assistants in the hospital to move to house companions' jobs. Our questions about the status of earnings were designed to see if we could gauge the relative significance of such differentials to the household. We expected a further gender difference. Almost all (94 per cent) of the men described their earnings as a major part of the household income, compared with 41 per cent of the women; another 41 per cent of the women described their earnings as a significant part. Only 10 per cent of the women talked of their salary as a minor part of the household income.

This matches the kind of response we obtained concerning promotion and career prospects. As we reported in Chapter Three, the staff in the community were not generally in the middle of the life-cycle and, putting all these facts together, we can suggest that the recruitment of qualified men is likely to remain problematic in the community, whilst the recruitment of older women may hinge on the possibility of reasonably paid, part-time work.

8   Training: Reactions and Needs

In this chapter we examine several aspects of training in the two different services and bring together evidence from other sections of this report about the identified training needs of staff. In the first section our concern is with those features of the situation which follow from the professional training of qualified nurses and from the experience of hospital staff moving to community employment. In the next section we examine in-service training provision for all staff in terms of its distribution, the factors which underlie demand for it, and some general outcomes. Finally, we turn to the issue of training needs in the two service environments.

Qualified nurses and others

Throughout this book we have made comparisons within the hospital designed to help locate the nature of the professional divide between qualified staff and others. We found this divide to be overlaid by the bureaucratic structure and noted the pivotal role of the villa managers. Putting the relevant findings together paints a clear picture of the qualified staff (Dingwall and Lewis, 1983). Since they had often had early contact with members of the client group the qualified staff were strongly career oriented, tended to be highly self-motivated, geographically mobile and with a developed sense of professional identity. They were adaptable and had a more optimistic view of the potential of the residents in their care than did their unqualified colleagues. Similarly they tended to favour community care more than did the nursing assistants.

In the organisational context the registered nurses were aware of the team effort involved in work on the villas and often, as a result, de-emphasised their professional status, typically according only a nominal responsibility to their position. In fact, of course, their position was crucial and their responsibility rather more than nominal, as our findings concerning their role adjustments confirmed. At registered nurse level the amount of Role Ambiguity rose considerably above the average and Role Conflict likewise began to increase amongst qualified staff, including enrolled nurses. Starting from the level of enrolled nurses, qualified staff perceived a less than average amount of support from their immediate supervisors, confirming the increased responsibility associated with their status.

Two kinds of change seem to be implied by the move of qualified staff into community employment. Firstly, there are changes in the nature of the role that people are expected to fill, and secondly, there are changes in the nature of the work. This raises the issue of the relevance of the skills imparted by nurse training and by hospital experience generally. Recognising the 'rapid developments in the care of people with mental handicap over the last decade' the English National Board recently redesigned the approved syllabus of training for the Registered Nurse for the Mentally Handicapped (English National Board, 1982). That new syllabus is based on the three principles that are reiterated by most regional strategy documents, namely the three principles of the Jay Committee Report. The syllabus envisages students gaining much of their practical experience in ways which 'reflect the changing emphasis in patterns of care' and thus they will experience helping 'people and their families in their homes and in community residential care as well as in hospital' (p.64). Given the date of the change in the training syllabus we could not expect to encounter many newly qualified staff who had experienced the changed training. In fact two of our respondents who currently worked in the community had trained at the time of changeover. We could only ask our interviewees what impressions they had of the changes and what they thought of them. There seemed to be general agreement that the training and its organisation were much improved. We could not systematically evaluate any changes associated with the newly implemented syllabus but we could ask about the perceived relevance of hospital based skills and about the mix of ex-hospital and non-hospital staff working in the staffed houses.

Firstly, we examined the role characteristics of community staff in terms of the measures employed in Chapter Five. In that chapter we noted the higher level of Role Ambiguity experienced by community staff. Closer examination showed that ex-hospital staff were responsible for most of the higher levels of Role Ambiguity amongst all community staff. Although the unqualified ex-hospital staff experienced the most Role Ambiguity, the average score of the qualified ex-hospital staff was still much higher than that of any group within the hospital ($p < .05$).

Perhaps the most interesting finding was that, within the community service, all the staff with hospital experience recorded much higher levels of Role Ambiguity than their colleagues who had had no such experience. The latter group still scored higher than nursing assistants, enrolled nurses and even charge nurses/sisters working in the hospital, but transferring to the staffed houses seemed to have produced a considerable confusion for hospital staff in terms of their role. Role ambiguity was also felt by qualified staff within the hospital, with registered nurses experiencing the highest levels. But confusion over authority, objectives and efficiency was greater amongst those who had moved to work in the staffed houses. One implication of these findings is that the hospital training of the staff had not fully prepared them for community work. Although the work situation was sufficiently blurred within the hospital to produce ambiguity, especially for registered nurses, the bureaucratic structure took some of the resulting strain and passed it up to villa management level. Some ambiguity is to be expected amongst professional staff, of course, since it reflects the need for expertise that generates the requirement for professional training in the first place. Clearly that requirement had changed for our respondents who had moved into the community. As we noted in

Chapter Six, the need for support was at its greatest for villa managers and this reflected the 'buck-passing system' that has been attributed to the hospital service (Felce, 1983). In the community, despite the degree of frustration evident in the level of autonomy that we reported, the staff were relatively more isolated and were expected to operate independently, to generate solutions and initiate actions in a manner consistent with the practitioner image of the nurse.

'There are so many more different demands on you in this job ... more than in the hospital. More decision making. There was nobody else to pass the buck on to. I did want more demands on me – but I found it difficult.'

For registered nurses moving to the community the most likely post is that of supervisor or home manager, or, as here, house co-ordinator. The extra strain of a first level of managerial responsibility adds to the confusion expressed over goals and produces even higher levels of uncertainty.

The second aspect of roles concerns Conflict. Again we saw the responsibility of qualified staff reflected in their higher levels of Role Conflict within the hospital. In the community it was ex-hospital staff who experienced the most Role Conflict, centred on the lack of resources (items 8, 13; see Questionnaire Appendix). This aspect of their role almost certainly reflected the relative lack of experience amongst hospital staff of having to seek resources for themselves. The community service management recognised the differential ability of hospital and other staff in this regard. Social workers were seen as having greater ability to seek out needed resources. On the other hand, nurses were more likely to have had some management experience, and in this they were valued by comparison with those from a social work background who were unlikely to have had such experience.

Within the hospital Role Conflict included not only such aspects as insufficient staffing levels, but also the frustration experienced by staff who could not implement the care practices of which their training made them aware. The English National Board, in its new syllabus, draws specific attention to the fact that comparison of care practices with the principles of normalisation, now taught as one of the core concepts in RNMH training, 'may lead to a conflict between theory and practice causing the student to experience marked cognitive dissonance' (English National Board 1982, p.18) Role Conflict is one manifestation of such dissonance in the staff.

'My experience is relevant [to community work] ... although it is quite a lot different. But when you work in a place like this you see ways in which you would like to improve things but under the system, in this set up, you can't. [Reference to training] Rather than being taught the things that we should be doing now – we are experiencing the things that we shouldn't be doing.'

(Charge nurse)

As we showed in Chapter Four, it was the more senior staff who were most likely to endorse the community care options; thus a degree of mismatch beween actual and prefered practice has long been a feature of the profession. The recognition by the English National Board of the problems such contradictions may raise for newly qualified people simply underlines the possibility that, as acceptance of the new care philosophies spreads, the degree of the mismatch may become greater. It is clearly the professional commitment of the qualified nurses which leads them to approve of the community service, even if they mostly draw the line at the level of the most dependent group of residents. If, as most published regional documents suggest, a group of highly dependent residents remain in hospital type provision, then the contradictions experienced by newly trained staff will have to be more sensitively addressed.

As we reported in Chapter Two, the proportion of newly qualified hospital staff recruited direct from the hospital school has dropped to about four in ten as staff take up community posts in preference. Those taking up hospital posts will benefit from any managerial and administrative experience but will increasingly encounter a hospital population that is much less able. Their own training, based on the new syllabus, will have emphasised non-institutional aspects of caring and the management of new staff will probably be more difficult as a result. The evidence from our research, and the increased responsibility generated by a new structure which provided only one villa manager, leaves little doubt that the role of villa manager will become even more critical as time passes. We will return to this issue later in this chapter.

It is the theory of normalisation which the English National Board indicates is likely to produce 'cognitive dissonance'. Describing her recent research Radford (1988) writes of a widespread need among care staff for information on normalisation and the philosophy of community care. As we found, when we examined beliefs in Chapter Four, for most staff in the hospital there was a correlation beween the degree of potential seen amongst residents and the strength of approval for community care options. We conclude that the type of care seen as appropriate was judged on the basis of presumed resident ability. This was in contrast to staff in the community, for whom the two measures were independent. Service options were not judged on the basis of ability and we concluded that the type of care seen as appropriate was mostly judged on the basis of residents' rights. Amongst qualified staff in the hospital the strength of this correlation was less than that amongst unqualified staff and at villa management level it was no longer significant. It is likely that newly qualified staff would be closer in their outlook to those now working in the community.

Those who had gone to work in the community service believed, as did the villa managers in the hospital, that the appropriate form of service for their clients was not ability-dependent. Disputes over the interpretation of normalisation were common in both organisations but were structured somewhat differently in each. In the hospital it was practical problems, and the message that they carried about general practicality, that were most often evidence of the conflict between current ideas and institutional constraints. The role of qualified staff in providing guidance to nursing assistants was highlighted many times by incidents which demonstrated that institutional values often guided the interpretation of events by nursing assistants who saw some of the changes as likely to fail as a result.

> 'In some ways they're going over the top now, going too silly with it all. Some of the things they're buying them, I feel their money is just squandered. Some of the things they buy are just unsuitable ... [The clothes] ... go down to the laundry and they're ruined. So we need someone to wash them in a washing machine and one thing follows another ... '

As the resident population reduces, and efforts are increased to prepare those remaining for community based care, such conflicts are likely to increase. To retain the co-operation of those for whom such changes are 'silly', for whatever reason, will put extra demands on the qualified staff.

In Chapter Four we characterised a number of staff as 'community-like' in their outlook. The proportion of nursing assistants who could be described in this way was of the order of 15 to 20 per cent of all unqualified staff. This group also shared with the qualified staff a separate view of residents' potential and service choice in that, for them, there was no relation between the two scales. For the rest of the unqualified staff there was, in contrast, a fairly strong relation. As closure approaches it is likely that there will be a reduction in the proportion of staff who have strongly positive attitudes towards community care. We may surmise, therefore, that the load on the qualified staff will increase still further. Since those with the most recent experience of training are the most likely to leave, it is the qualified staff who trained some time ago whose need for in-service training is likely to be greatest.

> 'All the staff on the ward were shocked by the Care Plan forms when they came round. We really do need study days for that sort of thing.'

We will return to the issue of appropriate in-service training in the next section, noting here that qualified staff who remain in the hospital during the run-down period will increasingly face extra demands.

If normalisation raised practical problems in the hospital, it was more often philosophical differences which arose in the community service. In the hospital, as we showed in Chapter Four, only a small proportion of nursing assistants were particularly 'community-like', so that qualified staff in general had more of a leadership task facing them. In the community all the staff shared very similar general views about care provision and were employed at the same level below the co-ordinator. The possibility of disagreement could therefore centre on the nature of staff's qualifications. What views did staff hold about the relevance of hospital experience? There were many different variations in the replies to those questions. Community staff with hospital experience tended to see that experience as providing a helpful introduction to community work; no one in the community described hospital training as fully relevant, and the usual response was a list of particular skills.

'[The RNMH] was useful in some ways but inadequate in others ... really very little of the hospital training was relevant ... ICPs were a useful background, at least I knew how to identify a teaching need and instigate a programme ... It took me months to get out of the routine of work [at the hospital].'

In fact it was usually the *pattern* of work experience, rather than the content of training, that qualified staff referred to when making negative comments about their own hospital backgrounds, and they were usually aware of this distinction, which is a direct reflection of the Role Conflict their hospital colleagues demonstrated in the survey:

'I felt that I couldn't practice what I learnt in the hospital but I could in the community. I did find it a bit difficult to adapt even though I had tried not to slip into the hospital habits.'

Most of the comments included positive remarks about some aspects of their experience, but when we collated all the kinds of reply under a simple 'positive, uncertain, negative' classification the professional division within the community appeared. In Table 8.1 this classification is shown for each of four groups, ex-hospital staff vs. others in the community and qualified staff vs. others in the hospital.

Table 8.1

Nature of comments about the value of hospital based skills to the community service (per cent of interview responses)

	Community ex-hospital	Community non-hospital	Hospital qualified	Hospital unqualified
Any positive remarks	75	14	67	38
Uncertain	—	—	11	62
Only negative remarks	25	86	22	—

Within the community the divide between the ex-hospital staff and others was quite clear. Again it was the general approach of the ex-hospital staff that other community staff tended to remark on in their comments:

'They were less sure of the hands off approach.'

The ex-hospital staff made comments in much the same way as their qualified colleagues in the hospital. There, the unqualified staff differed from all other groups in being very unsure of the situation. Radford (1987) reports a widespread uncertainty about the implications of community care. In our study it was clear that most qualified staff thought they understood some of the implications in terms of the relevance of their own skills, but unqualified staff generally had little notion of what might be implied.

What are the implications of these findings? Table 8.1 suggests that in the hospital qualified staff take the lead in terms of normalisation. But having and needing knowledge are rather different aspects of the situation. We will discuss the targeting of knowledge in the next section of this chapter, but we note that for the majority of nursing assistants anticipatory training for the community is related to the probability of their taking up such work. Most were not particularly oriented towards community employment and, furthermore, only a minority were particularly positive about community type service. In other words their uncertainty was only problematic to the extent that other services may wish to recruit them.

The results presented in Table 8.1 suggest a major source of stress within the service, but this would be to assume that the differences in background, which we have shown to be related to judgements about the appropriateness of skills, are also the basis for operational differentiation. In fact, this would almost certainly be an exaggerated response. We asked specifically about differences between the trained and untrained staff as a further check on this possible divide. An analysis of replies to these questions showed that, in operational terms, the divide was of little significance. For example, as many ex-hospital staff as others made comments which included negative remarks about the different approaches of trained or untrained staff, and there were the same number of staff making positive comments from both sorts of background. Such questions are also unfair in that we could not ask in the same way about the backgrounds of those with no relevant experience. In fact, of course, at the level of specific skills, the ex-hospital staff had very valuable expertise which was recognised by them-selves, their non-hospital colleagues and by the management. Differentiation within the staff tended to centre on the overall approach of the ex hospital staff and on 'institutional' practices. certainly there was no tendency for ex-hospital staff to be less optimistic about the residents' abilities. In fact, on our scales of resident *and* service orientation, the differences went the other way. Ex-hospital staff saw *more* potential in the residents than their colleagues, scoring higher by an amount that is unlikely to be due to chance ($p < .05$), and were *more* in favour of community service, though by a smaller margin ($p < .1$).

In most of the discussion above we have referred to 'ex-hospital' staff and not made the separation by qualifications. In fact, most of the ex-hospital staff were qualified; only two interviewees had worked as nursing assistants and their views were similar to those of their colleagues. One additional source of differentiation occasionally surfaced in the interviews which confirmed what we concluded about the distribution of views within the hospital. It was clear from their replies that people generally, but especially those in the community, considered that a proportion of staff were 'institutionalised'. We have shown that the great majority of staff in the hospital endorsed some form of community care but that a proportion of staff, mostly unqualified, based their view on notions of ability, rather than rights. We have argued that in practical terms most nursing assistants will probably not wish to pursue community employment. When staff from the two services co-operate and come into contact, misunderstandings seem likely to occur. This means that there should be careful development and management of links between hospitals that are running down, and the community services which are receiving their residents.

We conclude this section with a consideration of the nature of qualifications in the community service. At present there is no unified training that crosses the boundaries of social work and nursing expertise; thus there is no single specialist qualification. Inevitably young people recruited directly into a community service by a local authority will face competition for more senior posts from people with a suitable qualification. It would seem that nursing qualifications are numerically more likely at this time to fit that bill, though social work qualifications also apply. In our interviews we did encounter the dilemma that faces some unqualified staff. Those who are able and ambitious and who already have expertise in the community may recognise, and believe, that both professions contribute to the effective service but feel unwilling to opt for only one. It would seen better if such uncertainties could be resolved by joint qualification. Progress in this direction has been made, but has been slow (CCETSW 1986; GNC/CCETSW 1982).

In-Service Training, Provision and Reactions

Training of any kind is expensive. Its opportunity cost is high, especially where staff shortages are a problem, and such shortages are common in both of the services that we have examined. Many respondents confirmed the findings of Radford (1985) that staff shortage made training very difficult to organise. Training also adds to the already high cost of turnover (Baysinger and Mobley, 1983) so the efficient targeting of training is very important. Our first question in this part of the chapter, therefore, concerns who received some (in-service) training in the year before our survey. Table 8.2 gives the proportions within each staff group who had received any training in the period, and the average duration of training.

Table 8.2
Proportion of staff at each level having received some in service training in previous year and average duration in days (per cent)

	Proportion	Average duration in days
Nursing assistants	13.2	4.2
Enrolled nurses	18.8	6.3
Registered nurses	46.2	8.2
Charge nurses/sisters	35.3	6.6
Senior nurses and above	27.3	2.3
All Community staff	42.0	8.5

Most of this training went to day staff (82 per cent) who were working full time (79 per cent). In a given period, therefore, the greatest training priority is given to registered nurses and to charge nurses and sisters. Within the hospital a third (33.7 per cent) of all qualified staff had received some in-service training in the previous year.

In the new community service nearly half the staff had received training. The figure given in Table 8.2 refers to the induction training. Many staff did not receive this since, as the service grew, its resources were temporarily overstretched. Subsequently when the training and development officer post was created, funds for temporary staff release were obtained from the EEC Social Fund (Pahl and Roose, 1990).

Over time the proportion of hospital staff who have received some training will, of course, tend to increase as those with longer service have more opportunity to attend at least one course. We asked about a specific period in order to gauge the relative priorities and we excluded short service hospital staff receiving induction training to increase the contrast. Because longer service staff will have had more opportunities to go on courses we would expect those receiving training during the period to have generally been employed for less time. For qualified staff this was the case. Those who had had some training in the year had an average length of service of 5.7 years, compared with 10.6 years for those who did not receive training. This highlights one of the problems associated with training. Although it is necessary to develop the skills of new staff, for example with a post qualifying management course, those staff will generally be younger and much more likely to leave the organisation. We could not trace any effect directly linked to training in 'Propensity to Leave', thus we are not arguing that training contributed to staff leaving, but the Propensity to Leave of staff who had received some training was significantly higher just because they were younger ($p < .05$). This was not the case for nursing assistants.

We can illustrate this by reference to those staff who actually did leave the hospital in the eighteen months following the postal survey. Of those who had received some training 36.2 per cent subsequently left, of those who had not received training only 18 per cent had left. One of the benefits often attributed to training is that it reduces the tendency of staff to leave (Kenny et al, 1979). We could not trace such an effect in the hospital.

What, other than organisational needs, might predict the demand for in-service training? When we analysed our measure of 'Training Required' we found two factors that contributed to an increased requirement amongst qualified staff. The first reflected needs generated by the tasks themselves, in that staff reporting greater Feedback from their jobs were less likely to feel they needed training and vice versa. The second reflected individual advancement, in that staff with lower satisfaction with extrinsic rewards (money, security) wanted more training. These are the results of an analysis which controlled for the effects of other possible factors such as age. The contributions, or effects, of Feedback and Satisfaction were the same (Feedback $-.21$; Satisfaction Factor $4 - .21$) but their implications are very different since Feedback from the job could be altered independently of training. For example, improved task management and supervision might compensate and reduce the need for training.

A similar picture was found in the case of unqualified staff. Lack of Feedback was again the strongest factor predicting demand for training. For unqualified staff a demand for training was also associated with lower job satisfaction, but in their case lower satisfaction reflected a lack of opportunities for self development. Unqualified staff, having greatly reduced opportunities for advancement in the career sense, thought they required more training when they felt under-used. In addition, demand for training amongst unqualified staff was dependent on Resident Orientation and Role Ambiguity. The perceived need for training was greatest amongst those unqualified staff who experienced lower levels of Feedback, more Role Ambiguity, were less satisfied with aspects of their self-development and were more optimistic about resident potential (Feedback − .29); Resident Orientation − .26; Role Ambiguity − .18; Satisfaction Factor 1 − .17).

The last of these emphasises the differentiation we found amongst staff in terms of their orientation towards the residents and service types. The perceived need for additional training did not reflect resident orientation amongst qualified staff, who were part of a well defined career structure, but for unqualified staff this was an important element. We compared the amount of Training Required, by membership of the 'community-like' group and by qualifications. The measure of 'Training Required' (question 11) was scored from 1 to 4, where 1 meant 'no additional training' and 4 meant 'continuous updating'. The overall average score was 3.06, almost exactly equivalent to the box labelled 'quite a lot more'. Table 8.3 gives the average scores for each of the groups.

Table 8.3
The expressed need for additional training by orientation and qualifications

	Community-like hospital staff	All other hospital staff
Qualified	3.7	3.5
Not qualified	3.1	2.6

Higher scores indicate a greater need for training

The difference for qualified staff between orientations could be due to chance, but the difference shown for unqualified staff between orientations is not a chance effect ($p < .05$). Also the differences within the orientation categories (columns) are probably real effects ($p < .001$). In other words, whilst unqualified staff generally see less need for additional training, this is particularly so for those who do not share the model of residents and service options held by community staff and many senior staff at the hospital.

In a similar way we attempted to trace, at a general level, the effects of in-service training. Because we had asked about the job in terms of its basic dimensions, we could compare the impact of training on those dimensions for different groups. We expected to find some differences among staff who had received some in-service training during the previous year. We also expected further positive effects, given that training carries important consequences for morale and motivation (Kenny et al. 1979).

In fact the range of effects for qualified hospital staff was quite considerable. We cannot confirm that the differences we found were *caused* by the receipt of training in the previous year and were not merely consequences of the process of selection, but the differences are at least plausible outcomes of in-service training. For qualified staff there were the following differences between those who had received some training and those who had not:

They reported higher levels of	:	Feedback
and	:	Autonomy
Better defined	:	Task Identity
A greater degree of	:	Participation in decision making
More	:	Supervisor Support
More positive	:	Resident Orientation
Were more pro-community	:	Service Orientation

These results mean that staff who had received some in-service training during the previous year were significantly different from those who had not received any training. They were likely to feel they received more feedback about how they were doing their jobs, they reported more autonomy in doing them, and they felt they had a better idea of what the work required. They were more likely to feel that they took part in decision making and felt more positive about the support they received from their superiors. Finally, those who had received training had higher expectations of residents and were more positive about the development of a community-based service. Interestingly, the amount of additional 'Training Required' by those who had received some recent training was less than for those who had not ($p < .05$), and this complements the above range of effects by confirming that staff *recognised* the effectiveness of their training to some extent.

Not only did unqualified staff receive less training, and think that they required less further training to do their jobs, but the effects of the training they had received were minimal. The sole effect was on Task Identity. Those nursing assistants who had received some recent in-service training had a slightly better defined view of the way their job fitted into the service as a whole ($p < .05$).

In the community the training covered by our survey was almost exclusively limited to the induction course. The importance of some form of induction was recognised by the management team, who mounted and ran the courses themselves when the service was first set up. As we suggested in Chapter Three the induction period was a difficult time for staff and most publications dealing with the setting up of new community services emphasise the importance of an induction programe (Allen, 1983 p.40; Mansell et al. 1987; Ward, 1984). At the time of the survey about half the community staff had received the training and half not, so we had a good opportunity to compare the two groups of staff to check the effects the induction training had produced.

In terms of the job itself, those community staff who had received induction training described their job as being characterised by more Autonomy ($p < .05$); they saw it as better defined, in the sense of seeing how their job fitted into the service as a whole (Task Identity, $p < .05$); they experienced less Role Ambiguity ($p < .09$) and they had a lower Propensity to Leave ($p < .05$). In addition their orientation towards community employment, measuring their preference for where they would work if they had to leave, was more pro-community ($p < .05$).

Not only is this an indication of the effectiveness of the induction courses which were put on, it is also a warning about the need to ensure that community services are provided with adequate training resources. Quite apart from the levels of effectiveness in the work, which may be inferred from the differences in the job dimensions, the reduced Propensity to Leave is a clear indication of the value of an early induction programme. Perhaps of equal value is the related difference in Community Employment Orientation. As we found in our earlier analysis of the Propensity to Leave, those who were most likely to leave the hospital were not necessarily particularly oriented towards community employment. Training in the hospital had no effect on the orientation, which is perhaps not surprising. Some wastage to the service as a whole was therefore indicated. Amongst community staff, we see how an induction programme can be an effective way to reduce staff wastage. In a new service it would seem prudent to allow for training resources in advance of the first setting-up of units, in order to minimise the possibility of an intial high staff turnover.

Training needs

In the previous section, we deliberately kept the discussion at a general level. In this section our concern is with specific requirements. Our approach is two fold. Firstly, we asked staff to talk directly about the jobs they were expected to do and the skills they felt they needed to accomplish their tasks. Secondly, we inferred from our various analyses what appeared to be lacking in each setting.

The first thing we can note is that, in the interviews, a considerable number of respondents were unable to list any specific training requirements. There were very considerable differences between the community and hospital staff. Amongst the former, 88 per cent said that they needed some additional training, but amongst hospital staff this proportion was less than half. There was no difference between qualified and unqualified staff: 41 per cent of nursing assistants and 42 per cent of all qualified staff identified at least one specific training need. These findings complement those we have reported concerning the response of staff to their roles. Community staff, for example, had considerably higher Role Ambiguity. Furthermore both qualified and unqualified staff in the community service, from either hospital or other backgrounds, gave approximately the same listing of topics. Table 8.4 sets out the kinds of needs identified by qualified and unqualified hospital staff and all community staff. The only difference between qualified and unqualified staff within the community was with respect to the 'management' category; only one house companion mentioned this. The distribution of topics is similar to that found amongst nursing staff in the recent study by Radford (1985, p.138).

Although the job of nursing assistants in the hospital is facing some changes, for example, as the result of gradual moves towards more individual, resident-centred activities and away from basic custodial care, the job is still essentially that of basic care. Where they see a need, therefore, is in areas related to basic nursing care. Individual care plans were beginning

Table 8.4

Specific training needs identified by staff (numbers of times each item mentioned in interviews)

	Community staff	Qualified hospital staff	Unqualified hospital staff
Management skills	5	3	—
Medical care/first aid	—	1	4
Teaching skills	9	2	1
Behaviour modification/management	6	3	—
Updating on new approaches	—	1	4
Deinstitutionalisation	1	1	—

to feature in their work, but for most nursing assistants demands for the teaching of residents had not yet produced sufficient uncertainty for them to perceive a need for special training. However, some were aware of their lack of understanding of the rationale for many of the changes.

'I think it would be nice to get some sort of refresher course. Sometimes when you talk to the students you feel ... I don't know ... we just don't know how people are thinking. What's going on.'

Hence the expressed need for updating amongst the nursing assistants.

Among qualified staff in the hospital the parallel to the nursing assistants' concern with basic care is the nurses' demand for management training. This is a parallel demand because, like basic nursing care for nursing assistants, it is part of their normal role, but they will not necessarily have had sufficient training in it. The urgency of the need for first line management skills has been recorded in a national study of nurse training (Brown and Walton, 1984 p.208). We have already noted the value placed on these skills as a commodity in the community service. Inevitably, as the concentration of more dependent residents continues, the need for closer supervision of care work, and the addition of more resident training programmes and better defined care plans, will increase the demand for support in the managerial role. This will be most acute at the villa management level. Radford (1985 p.44) reports, in her national survey, that Directors of Nurse Education give the highest training priority to charge nurse/sisters. Certainly the findings which we summarized at the beginning of this chapter emphasise the crucial role of this level within the nursing hierarchy, and it is not surprising that all those who mentioned a need for training in management skills were at that level.

We also noted, in Chapter Five, the wider view of the nursing role that was displayed by staff at the villa management level. This wider view is reflected in Table 8.4 in the range of training needs from staff at this level. But, of course, any classification scheme such as this will separate out aspects of the topic which were in reality part of an overall view. As one staff member said,

'I would definitely need some kind of a refresher course [to function in the community] – my training was a long time ago and I'm institutionalised now. Working in the hospital, we just start one routine and

finish another one, but working in the community you're based on
a different level. Training a resident to do cooking, for example, that
rarely happens here as yet. Because the staff level is so poor, we just do the
basic things for them.'

(Charge nurse)

As Table 8.4 showed, training needs, for example in the teaching of skills,
were matched by needs relating to behaviour management. When the
proportion of more able residents was higher, training effort was concentrated on those residents. As the proportions have begun to change, more
and more of the residents with challenging behaviour have been brought
into the instruction programmes. Staff, who had not had special instruction in teaching techniques, reported to us the additional difficulties that
this caused.

What were still anticipatory demands in the hospital, though of growing
urgency, were by contrast everyday needs amongst community staff.
Where staff had had some prior experience of the teaching of skills, for
example in a training unit at the hospital, they felt some confidence
in the task. Similarly some community staff reported the value of their
nurse training in specific areas such as behaviour modification techniques,
preparation of care plans and even teaching techniques. However, the
majority of staff, including those from hospital backgrounds, felt insuf-
ficiently skilled in the areas of behaviour management and teaching. It is
interesting to note that precisely these two areas were identified as
specific needs by staff in the Wells Road service in Bristol, six months after
a thorough induction training (Ward, 1985). With only a small number
of residents to focus upon and a large number of teaching objectives, the
community staff were acutely aware of their performance. The first few months
following the discharge of a resident usually produced a highly visible
change in appearance and behaviour, and the staff were well aware of these
changes. Those from hospital backgrounds spoke of the value of having
witnessed the hospital conditions, since it provided them with a useful baseline;
they felt they understood what residents faced in leaving the hospital.
Within the first year, however, the improvement rate for residents was considerably reduced and staff were much less sure of their impact. We have
recorded the universally low levels of feedback described by staff. Given
the goals of the community service, it is a paradox that, as resident potential
is realised and residents' abilities increase, the job becomes more demanding
of staff skills in the area of training, simply because the gain in a given time
needs a more developed professional eye to record it. Continuing in-
service training is an essential component of any service which seeks to
develop the full potential of its clients.

In the community the disruption caused by those residents who exhibited
behaviour problems could have widespread effects. We have recorded
the impact of broken 'sleep-in' shifts on staff stress, but unco-operative
behaviour from a single resident could prevent organised activities in
the house, such as shopping trips. So, quite apart from the benefits to the
individual resident, more effective behaviour management is necessary

for the improved quality of life of all clients, given that segregation is not an option.

Finally, the community staff, both house companions and house co-ordinators, wanted more management training. These were, as we have reported, ambitious people, and they were aware of the value of management experience. Getting some training was of personal value to them but, in addition, the running of a staffed house had put a strain on the house co-ordinators, especially at first, and some form of first line management experience was obviously of considerable value (c.f. Ward, 1984).

In this section, we have reported expressed needs for training; can we add specific areas that seem indicated by other responses from staff? It would be valuable to have some clarification, especially in the induction training, with respect to Normalisation. This, of course, is a developing concept (Wolfensberger, 1972; 1980) which is linked to an evaluation procedure for care environments (Wolfensberger and Glenn, 1975; Wolfensberger and Thomas, 1983 and see Tyne and O'Brien, 1981). Some of the community staff had attended a course on this, but we encountered considerable variations in the interpretation of the ideas behind the approach. The misunderstanding that it is to do with 'normality', in the sense of 'conformity' (Mansel et al. 1987), was present in the replies of several staff. Furthermore, several staff felt that the uncertainty concerning it was widespread.

> 'It means something different to everybody I think.' 'Everyone has their own ideas about it. At the meeting we had this silly long conversation about the bed linen, because people had their own ideas about what was the more 'normal' thing to do.'

Whilst such disputes may be quite proper in a professional sense, the confusion we encountered was clearly the result of a lack of understanding of the principles involved. Disputes around the theme of normalisation echoed the division between ex-hospital staff and those from other backgrounds. Appropriately focussed induction training would probably reduce this, as would the existence of some joint qualification.

What conclusions can we draw from our findings about the form and targetting of in-service training? Staff responding to Radford's regional survey (1985) suggested that staff trained in specific areas could be trained to be effective in passing on skills informally. We found such informal instruction within the community service with respect to management development, and between staff at the same level who taught one another the basics of the co-ordinators job. However, given the dearth of expertise in resident instruction skills, and in the management of behaviour, and bearing in mind our conclusion about staff motivation, some direct training input in these areas would be valuable. The development of training is obviously limited by available resources. Equally the scale of provision has an impact on the limits of informal instruction and staff development. In the community service staff were expected to be individual practitioners, rather than basic caretakers. Within the context of a staffed house, there were likely to be few staff with high levels of expertise in the areas where training was wanted, so more formal training was necessary.

The situation is slightly different in the hospital, where the scale is larger and there is a well developed training department. Even so the limitations of staffing and training resources in a reducing service make the efficient use of existing expertise of even greater importance. Two conclusions follow from this. Firstly, the informal training function of qualified staff could be enhanced by ensuring that qualified staff receive appropriate in-service instruction; this study has shown the wide range of effects on those who had received any recent in-service training. Secondly, as so many of our findings indicate, it is the villa management level that is critical in the hospital. The more effective management of staff in the advanced stages of a reduction and/or closure programme demands the development of management skills at this level.

Conclusions

In this final chapter we discuss the findings of our research in terms of the implications for services. It is always difficult to know how much to generalise from any one study, especially in a period of rapid change, but this book, and the research on which it is based, focusses on the two major changes likely to have future relevance: the reduction and closure of NHS long-term hospital provision and the development of local authority community services. The clear trend towards a reduction in large NHS provision and the growth of local authority services are both now likely to continue at enhanced rates following the Government's acceptance of the Griffith recommendations.

Some of the implications for staffing in the future services will almost certainly echo the processes we examined. For example, from the outset, the new community service attempted to recruit staff who would be age and gender appropriate for its clients. It had some success in this, achieving over 40 per cent male staff, but maintaining this proportion would seem to be problematic. The community service found it difficult to recruit staff in the age range from 30–44 years. Simple explanations based on pay levels have some validity, but in the hospital this age band was well represented. We found that women with children were more likely to work night shifts and to be part-time, and we traced 15 different combinations of hours which were being worked within the hospital, in addition to the basic shifts. A quarter of the staff were part-time employees, but their employment history, measured as length of service, showed that they made a major contribution to the stability of the hospital service. At a time when widespread concern is being expressed in the nursing service as a whole we feel it is important to emphasise this point. Women working part-time had suited their hours to their domestic circumstances and, as a result, had worked on average many *years* more than full time staff. Managements everywhere should take note that part-time staff, who are often marginalised by organisations, are, at least in this one way, a *more* valuable resource than many short service, full time employees. One way in which a community service could both improve the proportion of employees in the middle age range and increase the stability of its workforce over time would be to find ways of employing women with dependent children for part-time hours.

The choice of shift arrangements has other implications. In the community service night cover was provided by a 'sleep-in' arrangement. Continuity of care was ensured by having the same people working during the two days on either side of a sleep-in shift. A single disruptive incident involving a resident at night could have a major impact on the performance of the staff person during the following day. The requirement for evening and night cover, and the lack of part-time or flexible arrangements, severely limited the number and types of people willing and/or able to work in the service. Given the small scale of the houses as units, and the difficulties experienced by staff facing pressure from very long shifts, it would seem reasonable to provide for additional flexibility in staffing arrangements. In the hospital cover for short-staffing situations could be found from other units because of the scale of operation. In the community, a part-time and flexible source of staff would alleviate the problems of staff absence.

Finding sufficient male staff is more problematic, especially in the middle age ranges. Typically men do not seek part-time work and the salary range available implies that few men with dependents will be likely candidates. Younger men will only be retained if the career structure is adequate. Within the local authority service this may imply some movement away from the client group. The community staff we studied had more flexible individual career strategies than the hospital staff, reflecting a more fluid response to occupational opportunity; one third did not intend to remain with the client group. It is possible that a specialist qualification would change this proportion.

The community service had recruited staff from both nursing and social services backgrounds. They were all highly motivated and committed to the ideals behind community care. There was no indication that those with hospital experience were any less committed; indeed they were actually more positive in their view of resident potential and had marginally greater faith in the community ideal. Most community staff were local people, but they were potentially much more geographically mobile than the average for the hospital. Furthermore most anticipated fairly immediate career improvements. They were ambitious and, since the opportunities within one service could not meet all such expectations, their retention was a problem. A service staffed largely by highly committed positive and ambitious young people is fundamentally unstable, and this will be reflected in high turnover rates. An adequate induction course might alleviate some of this but the employment of staff with different motivations, working on a part-time basis, or with lower self-development needs, ought to increase long term stability.

In general we found that the beliefs of community staff were similar to those of registered nurses, villa managers and nursing officers within the hospital but different from most nursing assistants. With respect to resident potential only nursing officers shared the degree of belief in community care that we found amongst community staff. However, attitudes towards community care were subtly different in the two organisations. In general community staff saw care in the community in terms of residents' rights, whilst in the hospital it tended to be judged in terms of practicality based on residents' abilities.

Nearly half of the community staff, despite very strong support for these ideals, believed it likely that a minority of clients would always require special provision. Indeed the only factor we could trace which *reduced* community staff commitment to the new service was the reported proportion of behaviour problems. Although the hospital staff tended to see the minority needing special provision as quite large, this was an area of agreement between the two sets of staff. Given the need for both types of organisation to co-operate at many levels, both services would benefit from knowing that some form of community care is supported by most hospital staff and some needs for special provision are recognised by most community staff. Disagreement seems likely to centre on the basic mis-understanding of rights versus practicality. Given the widespread plans for special provision, the proposed services for the more challenging residents should be given a higher profile to provide an anchor for the views of staff and to make clear the scope of the proposed changes.

Beliefs about community care were linked to the hospital staffs' beliefs about their own likely role. Many feared an anti-nurse feeling in the community. In our view, and in the experience of the community service we studied, these fears were unfounded. We have argued that there is a certain absurdity in the idea that whilst residents can be discharged and de-institutionalised all their former professional caretakers can be viewed as unsuitable employees because they have become 'institutionalised'. An adequate induction and orientation course is what is required.

Not all hospital staff will necessarily want to transfer to the community services or be easily able so to do. Because the ex-hospital staff in the community were a self-selected group, we used their responses as a model and found about a fifth of the hospital staff with a similar outlook. These people were either senior qualifed staff, older, less mobile and less likely to leave than average, or they were young, mobile staff who were very likely to leave. We traced a process by which staff with less progressive views were being concentrated within the hospital, but noted that senior staff were usually in the vanguard with respect to views of the new service options. We concluded that the role of senior staff, especially at villa manage-ment level, will become increasingly demanding as the service runs down and this process continues. We felt it especially important that their long term commitment to the client group, and their obvious advocacy of alternative forms of care, should be recognised and understood by those seeking their co-operation in the development of those new forms of care.

We have already noted the different shift systems in operation and the opportunities for different working arrangements. Both organisations also relied on overtime working but there was considerably more of this in the community. We suggested that part-time working in the community might be one way to offset staff shortage but part-timers in the hospital, and probably in general, were unable to work overtime to the same degree, and this would undoubtedly be true in the case of voluntary over-time, which we found exceeded three hours per week in the community. As much flexibility in hours as possible is therefore indicated.

The actual organisation of work in the two settings was, of course, very different. To gauge staffing levels, employers usually quote the ratio of staff to residents. However, we would suggest that the number of staff usually available at any given time is a better guide to the actual situation being faced. In the community the crucial figure is *one* member of staff. The major determinant of activity outside the staffed houses is the presence of more than one staff person. It is this that permits outside 'community' contact. The level of dependency and the proportion of behaviour problems in the community was reported to be lower than in the hospital but a single disruptive individual can have a disproportionate effect within a staffed house. Various strategies for isolating and containing problems, which could be pursued in the hospital, were impossible in the staffed houses. The results could be harmful both for staff and for other residents. This highlights the need for additional help, especially in the area of behaviour management, for the existing staff in the houses. One possibility, which would take account of the variations between houses, would be to ensure organisational flexibility by having different shift arrangements where frequent night disruption occurs.

The nature of the work in the hospital revolves around the villa as a unit. There is a major change in the way people describe their job at the charge nurse/sister level with the managerial role predominating. This is not surprising in itself but, crucially, the level of reported resident interaction was at its highest at this grade. The type of interaction described by staff was also qualitatively different at this grade than at all others, being much more actively resident-centred. The style of activity on a villa is effectively decided at that level and our analysis showed that the level of role conflict experienced by charge nurses and sisters was the highest in the hospital. General managerial responsibility was increasingly difficult at this level, as villa managers attempted to cope with staff shortages and introduce new care practices. Putting these findings together identifies the villa managers as the most critical staff grade in a reducing hospital.

We have argued that charge nurses/sisters should be the prime targets for managerial support and training initiatives within the hospital, recognising that their role is changing from one of basic administration to one of much more active management. We found that basic care staff, especially nursing assistants, who form the backbone of the service, expressed minimal role ambiguity and conflict. They believed they knew very well what their role actually was. In this they were not entirely correct. As the resident population becomes more dependent, and the typical form of care increasingly involves training rather than merely containing the clients, the role of the care staff will constantly evolve. Clearly it will fall primarily to villa managers to oversee and guide this redefinition of the staff role. Adequate and *advance* preparation of the managerial skills required at charge nurse/sister level should therefore be a very important part of a reduction programme.

In the community, the nature of the work was different in several important ways. Community staff were quite isolated in the houses, but no more so than the average nursing assistant. They did report much higher levels of interaction with individual residents, although the average level was not significantly greater than that reported by charge nurses. However, their autonomy was on a par with that reported by nursing assistants and they reported similar levels of task variety and identity. This shows that the community staff did not have a significantly improved grasp of the way their job fitted in with the complete service provided for the residents. However, they did feel confident about the tasks involved in their own jobs.

Staff in both organisations were equally likely to think that planned goals existed for the job. However, when it came to how people fitted operationally into the organisation for achieving those goals, it was clear that the community staff experienced a situation that required a higher level of professional input. This was revealed by a very much greater degree of role ambiguity amongst community staff. Some increase in ambiguity is to be expected, given the broader professional span, but the difference was large enough to suggest that many staff found their role problematic. Clearly adequate training is required to improve staff confidence, given that narrower job definition and/or organisational control would be both self-defeating and against the 'anti-institutional' ethos of most community services.

Performance feedback was experienced as very low by all groups of staff, and this was as true in the community as in the hospital. Whilst performance review was defined as ineffective by most staff, direct feedback was seen as almost absent. There was one major exception to this. Many community staff had witnessed quite dramatic changes in the residents following discharge from hospital. This experience had positive effects on the outlook of other staff, but after the initial change, it was clear that staff could not easily see further progress. Only carefully targeted training can enhance the ability and confidence of staff to maintain programmes with residents, when the effects are slow to materialise.

The overall levels of perceived hierarchy and of participation by staff in the two organisations were similar, but typical responses to the way the two organisations operated were different. In the community problems were largely individual and professional, whilst in the hospital they were most frequently bureaucratic. In the hospital responsibility was attributed to rather neutral agents like 'the system' while in the community the service management was relatively more visible. The difference was probably due to the relative scale of the two services and highlights again the need for the confidence that training and/or good experience can provide.

Another consequence of scale is that, while in the hospital additional resources were likely to be made available at times of extra need, in the community the management team had to supply direct support as the service got under way. This carried an ambiguous message to staff about their competence. We stressed the importance of a strong commitment from the local authority from the outset, so that new services are not forced to rely on unrealistic levels of performance from staff. This means not only adequate management resources and basic staff, but the possibility of access to a pool of expert help, especially in the field of behaviour management.

We extended our analysis of organisational factors to include higher levels of authority. Two findings were of significance. In the community, the effective operational unit was the individual house. The staff in the houses made a very clear separation between their immediate service management team, the area social services and the county-wide local authority. However, the local authority bureaucracy interacted with the houses at a number of points in a way which suggested some confusion over the level of effective control vested in the new service. Clear and unambiguous decentralisation of functions such as greater budgetary control to the individual houses would probably be the best way of addressing this sort of problem.

In the hospital, staff placed the responsibility for low morale and similar problems at district and regional levels, with not much separation seen between the two. This has important implications for the management of hospital closure. The management of morale implies the need for a clear resolution of uncertainty at the strategic level as early as possible in a closure programme. One aspect of this is the need for health authorities to emphasise the *transition* of care services rather than simply presenting a closure plan for a particular institution. The latter leads to an institutional myopia and focusses people's minds on a supposed reduction of opportunities rather than what is, in effect, an expansion of services.

Within the hospital the management of closure is primarily concerned with the villas as units. For most staff the closure lacks impact because of its relative remoteness. The effects on staff are tied very closely to the villa closure schedule. In so far as possible, therefore, the implications for staff should be presented well in advance. Any organisational mechanism which allows staff to detach psychologically from a given unit in advance of its actual closure would help to maintain morale and retain staff. For example, allocating staff to their next location well before villa closure and 'loaning' them back, would help to reduce the uncertainty that is otherwise rife.

In a more general way, the employment opportunities within other agencies should be as visible as possible. The internal labour markets of the health service and of local authorities remain relatively closed. Joint working should include the effective dissemination of job vacancy information where this is relevant. The hospital should recognise the widespread effect of low morale on the local labour market, which is informally in contact with the service. Further recruitment is made more difficult when disaffection is spread by staff who may have no immediate intention of leaving themselves. Potential wastage to the service as a whole may result, as a small proportion of the most recent recruits to the closing hospital move on and take their experience to jobs in the community.

Professional organisations and unions are well established within the health service. One finding of our research, which may or may not mirror a widespread trend, is that the move to community care had resulted in lower levels of staff representation. There was a slight tendency for community staff to be less sure of the value of staff associations but, in general, it was a combination of apathy and poor organisation on the part of staff associations that was responsible for the very low membership. However, the potential for problems requiring professional protection remains in the new service, and was recognised by staff. Established staff associations should take note of this new situation.

How did staff satisfaction differ between the two services? Firstly, we noted that community staff were slightly better off in terms of income and consequently were slightly more satisfied with that aspect of the job. However, the relative differential between the residential social worker scale and the nurses' pay scale changed during the period of the study. Thus our finding was highly contingent and the situation is unlikely to be resolved by anything other than a redefinition of grades.

The community staff were rather less satisfied than the hospital staff with the number of hours they had to work. Inevitably the development of a new service put extra strain on staff, who worked additional hours overtime. The shift system added to the load, in that the 'sleep-in' tended to reduce the psychological separation of the day shifts, so that staff felt they were 'at work' for the whole period, even if their sleep was not disrupted.

The most significant components of job satisfaction were what we have labelled self-development aspects. Community staff were much less satisfied with these aspects of the job, which might be termed the 'challenge factor' of the work. However, this is not to say that the job was intrinsically less challenging. Indeed some of the evidence we have presented would suggest the reverse: for example, the degree of task variety was the same as that reported by charge nurses and sisters in the hospital and the amount of reported individual resident interaction was the highest we recorded. The most likely explanation for our finding relates to the available labour market and the motivation of staff. Since most community staff were young, mobile and highly motivated, they were much less likely to be satisfied with any given level of work. We found that their dissatisfaction with self-development was related to task variety and role ambiguity, so that the community staff who were the least satisfied perceived the least variety and the most ambiguity. Thus the situation could be remedied by appropriately focussed training and supervision. However, dissatisfaction is also a consequence of employing staff that are uniformly highly motivated. The appointment of some staff with lower self-development needs would not necessarily compromise the effectiveness of the service, given appropriate support and supervision, but would almost certainly improve its stability.

We expected that if the difficulties experienced by staff were sufficiently strong, they would appear as evidence of stress. The two organisations produced very similar levels of stress, according to our measurements, and we concluded that in general caring for people with mental handicaps, in either type of setting, was moderately stressful. We found values which suggested the job is more stressful than most other occupations, though still much lower than the values which have been found amongst parents caring for mentally handicapped children at home.

However, the causes of stress in the two services were rather different. When we interviewed staff we collected a list of stress-inducing pressures which staff could readily bring to mind. In the community staff mentioned the quantity of work, pressure from management, and the sleeplessness due to disturbed nights followed by day shifts. Some people complained of an atmosphere of 'intensity' in the houses, but this seemed to be an attribute of the staff, in the sense that so many were young and highly committed, motivated people. In the hospital the prevalence of behaviour problems caused stress, as did staff shortages, the quantity of work and the uncertainty associated with the hospital closure. We have already suggested that the community service would benefit from some extra flexibility in staffing and from the provision of at least some additional staff, who could provide cover for absence and/or nights. In the hospital we have argued that the resolution of uncertainty can only be accomplished by early and clear policy statements *effectively* disseminated and by advance notification of the re-allocation of staff at villa level. Many members of staff were appreciative of the regular briefings set up by the clinical services manager.

However, the factors which people can identify in free recall will not necessarily be those that contribute the most to stress. When we analysed our measure of stress we found two different patterns which fitted in with several of the comments which staff made about the nature of their jobs. In the community stress was related most strongly to role ambiguity and autonomy. Being left to cope with a poorly understood role accounted for much of the stress in the houses. In the hospital it was rather role conflict and the lack of individual resident interaction that produced an effect. Frustration in the community was produced by staff feeling uncertain about their expanded professional role. In the hospital it was produced by staff feeling unable to do the job in the way advocated by professional training and ideology. We noted the English National Board's warning that students would experience the contradictions between theory and practice as 'cognitive dissonance' and argued that pressure to change the form of care in the reducing hospital would produce similar effects amongst staff.

The practical implications were similar in both organisations but the balance was different. In the community resolution of the problem of ambiguity cannot be achieved simply by increased job definition, for two reasons. First, the new philosophy of care emphasises client-led initiative and open-endedness; secondly, increased job definition and more detailed supervision would reproduce the 'institution-like' qualities of the hospital service. The more productive solution, therefore, is an increase in appropriate training and support. Support was thought to be lacking by the majority of community staff. An increase in the scope of the professional role, reflected in greater ambiguity, is bound to generate some additional needs for 'support', but we found that staff were uncertain about how much backing they could expect. An intermediate managerial level was required at a fairly early stage to meet the needs of individual house co-ordinators. In the absence of this layer the service managers were the only people available to co-ordinators and we observed the self-defeating problems produced by their intervention, which despite being requested was nevertheless resented. Adequate resources for initial induction training for house co-ordinators or similar supervisors is obviously a priority for new services of this kind. Adequate support, in the form of flexible, excess staff capacity is another. The responsibility for arranging staff cover, especially for emergencies, should be clearly defined and, preferably, be based on the availability of a pool, so that houses are not forced to 'trade' staff.

In the hospital the level of perceived support showed a significant divide at villa management level, and this reinforced what we said about the pivotal role of this grade. The increased span of control of the villa managers, and the evolution of care practices for a gradually more dependent population will put increasingly heavy demands on charge nurses and sisters. All the qualified staff expressed some dissatisfaction with the levels of support they received. Apart from the obvious resource implications caused by staff absence this dissatisfaction revealed both the responsibility of the job and the limitations to the confidence people have in accomplishing it. We have already remarked on the fact that nursing assistants saw their job as being well defined. We argued that this was a misapprehension on their part. We also found that they saw little need for extra support. This too, paradoxically, is unlikely to be the case. As their job becomes more demanding, their need for support will increase. We have suggested that it will fall to villa managers to provide this, and that they should therefore be the prime targets for training resources, closely followed by other qualified staff.

We also found that the factors which caused stress in the community were also related to the propensity of staff to leave the service. Thus the new professional role was proving unacceptable to some staff. The propensity to leave, like the actual turnover, was slightly higher amongst community staff, but they were mostly young and mobile people anyway. Hospital staff were less likely to leave, having relatively more invested in the job and area. Consequently the main factors predicting propensity to leave in the hospital were age and job satisfaction, with younger and more ambitious staff being more likely to leave in a given period. The role of stress should not be overemphasised in the context of the community setting, since the overall level we recorded was similar to that in the hospital. It was just that the staff in the community were more able to *react* to that level of stress because they were more mobile. A more stable workforce would probably absorb the same level of stress.

Staff who left the hospital did not usually plan to work in the community service. We could not trace the destinations of ex-hospital staff but we did ask about intentions. One third of the staff said that they did not intend to remain with the client group. This was a little surprising and may constitute a further argument in favour of a more specialist qualification. Such a qualification might increase long-term commitment to serving people with mental handicaps.

The intentions of many hospital staff were best described as occupational inertia. Some had calculated that they could 'see the job out' in the hospital; others had recognised that community work would increase in availability and saw no immediate rush. The lack of obvious longer term prospects in the hospital meant that recruitment was more likely to become the major problem for the management, whilst in the community it was long term retention that seemed more problematic. We discovered that only about 17 per cent of hospital staff were considering community employment at the time of our research. This figure will probably increase as closure approaches. Among nursing assistants about 15–20 per cent would seek community employment.

We have shown that ex-hospital staff were suitable employees in the community service, but that pay differentials and different conditions might be a source of problems. The highly committed staff in the community service had, in some cases, been prepared to lose money in the job change, but the overall picture was, at that time, one of gain. The critical differential was at registered nurse level and this currently favours those employed by the health service. We have noted the fear of some hospital staff that they will not be welcomed into community employment but what aspects of their experience might add to or detract from their suitability?

In general ex-hospital staff had been readily employed by the community service but when we analysed this group, we found that they experienced the highest levels of role ambiguity. They also recorded the highest levels of role conflict, centred on lack of resources. The community management team believed that staff with social work backgrounds had more experience in finding resources, such as voluntary drivers and so on, which is a plausible explanation for this difference. Thus there was clearly something lacking in their experience.

The expanded professional role in the community is much closer to the 'practitioner' image of the nurse. Both the nature and the scale of the community houses intensify the feeling of independent responsibility in staff, especially at supervisory level. The increase in managerial responsibility at villa level was producing a similar effect in the hospital, and we predict that this will increase.

Though ex-hospital staff might lack experience in obtaining resources in the community they did tend to have managerial experience. This was a valued commodity in the new service. Even so 'management' was one of the topics mentioned by community staff as a training requirement. Given the youth and ambition of the typical community employee, this need was understandable. However, existing training resources cannot be expected to cope with such a level of demand. Management training, as an aspect of staff development, would need to be effectively targetted.

The ex-hospital staff who worked in the community service could bring their knowledge to bear, but there was some feeling that the daily pattern of their work reflected a different practice. Specifically, whilst the ex-nurses had skills in areas of identifying teaching needs, implementing programmes and, to some extent, managing behaviour, the ethos of the new service involved a 'hands off approach' that their colleagues felt they did not always understand. As might be expected, the specialist skills of the ex-nurses were mostly lacking in the staff from a social work background. However, both groups identified the same main areas of training need. The most prominent of these were resident teaching techniques, and behaviour modification and management.

In addition to these areas of training, our analysis suggested a need for some clarification in the area of normalisation theory. Ideological disputes over interpretation will obviously not disappear but a more developed understanding could be achieved with appropriate training. We were able to demonstrate a wide range of effects due to the induction training of community staff. Those who had had that training experienced less ambiguity, saw better how they fitted into the service and were less likely to consider leaving.

The relative independence and autonomy of community staff, coupled with the non-custodial model of care, suggested that they should all receive basic training, especially in teaching skills to residents. Behaviour management is the other area where most staff would benefit, although the possibility of obtaining additional outside expert advice in this area might constitute a better use of resources. However, all staff should receive an induction programme. This would present an opportunity for the principles of normalisation to be more uniformly spread. In addition any ex-hospital staff would benefit from a specifically designed re-orientation element which should aim to remove the label of 'institutionalised', which in our view is not a serious hurdle.

In the hospital, staff identified the same training needs, but it was mostly qualified staff who expressed those needs. We have already argued that efficient targetting implies that villa managers and registered nurses should be the recipients of the training resources. We were able to trace a wide range of effects of in-service training on the qualified staff, who benefited by gaining a more positive resident orientation and a better understanding of their role in the service. Benefits to nursing assistants were limited to slightly better job definition. Training in the hospital should give priority to management techniques, especially for villa managers, with the expectation that teaching skills and behaviour management will be passed on to nursing assistants by qualified staff who might, as part of their development, be taught more effective staff instruction techniques.

It was also clear that most staff, and this really means the majority of nursing assistants, were unclear about the new philosophy of care. The arguments enshrined in most regional strategy documents concerning residents' rights were not generally recognised or understood by unqualified staff. The effective management of uncertainty during a closure programme should therefore include more than advance warning of the implications for staff and their jobs. Staff need to understand *why* the policy has been decided, or they will react cynically and morale will fall. Briefing sessions about a closure programme could be complemented with presentations on the philosophy of care, which would not constitute large demands on resources. The benefits would be great, both for staff and for residents.

Appendix 1

This Appendix contains statistical details of the scales used in the research, a copy of the postal questionnaire and a copy of the interview checklist.

Postal questionnaire scales

1. *Performance and reliability*

The postal questionnaire appears in full at the end of this section. Here we report on the performance of the scales over the full response from the community and the hospital populations. Values for the full response on each item for the various scales are given in the reproduced questionnaire. In each case the first column gives the item mean, the second the item standard deviation and the third the corrected item-total correlation. These values are based on cases with no missing items for the particular scale and thus the number of respondents varies slightly between scales and is also reported.

2. *Treatment of missing data*

The number of responses on each scale is always sufficient for adequate analysis of a given scale, but for most multi-variable analyses a case missing on only one scale is deleted from the full treatment. This can result in a rapid drop in the total number of cases available for a detailed analysis. The bulk of missing cases, however, were missing on only one or two items in a given scale. To alleviate the problem these missing data were replaced by the overall means for those items. Only when the number of items missing on a given scale exceeded 20 per cent of the possible number was a case defined as invalid for that scale.

The reliability coefficients (Alpha) and factor structures reported for the scales in this section are based on fully valid cases, with no missing items, so that overall scale values may vary slightly from those reported in the main text of the report.

3. *Employment intentions*

Two scales tap these intentions: 'community employment orientation' (COMEMP) and 'propensity to leave' (PROLEVE). COMEMP comprises questions 16 and 17 on the questionnaire. These were each scored 1–4 ('not very …' = 1), so that the scale range is 2–8. The overall mean was 5.35, standard deviation was 1.81 and the two items gave Alpha = .60, a similar reliability to that in the pilot survey.

PROLEVE comprises the two items of question 31. These were each scored 1–5 ('never' = 1), giving a scale range of 2–10. The overall mean was

5.74, standard deviation was 2.42 and Alpha = .76; an improvement on the pilot results.

4. *Job satisfaction*

The 17 items of question 26 were scored 1–5 ('dissatisfied' = 1), giving a scale range of 17–85. The overall mean was 59.8, standard deviation was 9.78 and Alpha = .84.

A principal-components analysis yielded four factors for job satisfaction (JOBSATEX). These are used in the main analysis and are discussed in the main text of the report. Details of the (VARIMAX) rotated structure matrix are reported below. Only values for the coefficients of .4 and above are reported.

Item number (of question 26)	Factor 1 (self-development)	Factor 2 (convenience/ friendship)	Factor 3 (status)	Factor 4 (extrinsic rewards)
1	—	—	.41	.58
2	—	—	—	.77
3	—	.71	—	—
4	—	.84	—	—
5	—	—	—	.54
6	—	—	.44	—
7	—	.52	—	—
8	.45	—	—	.41
9	—	—	.76	—
10	.68	—	—	—
11	.80	—	—	—
12	.79	—	—	—
13	.75	—	—	—
14	.77	—	—	—
15	.74	—	—	—
16	—	—	.52	—
17	.62	—	—	—
Per cent explained variance	31.7	9.1	8.1	6.7

The scores for each respondent used in the analysis are based on the full values for each factor but the labels reflect the contributions made by those items loading most strongly on a given factor. Factor 4, for example, loads on items referring to pay, security, travel and promotion and is labelled 'Extrinsic rewards'.

5. *MALAISE*

The 24 items of question 25 were scored 1 'yes' and 0 'no', giving a range of 0–24. The overall mean was 2.62, standard deviation was 2.77 and Alpha = .75. The MALAISE scale is a measure of generalised health stress.

6. *Job dimensions*

The 12 items of question 27 measure six different dimensions of the job and were scored 1–5 ('very little' = 1). Each dimension is measured on a scale from 2–10, comprising two items which appear as separated pairs, as shown by the key in the reproduced questionnaire. The dimensions and their performance were as follows:

Name	Item pair	Scale mean	Standard deviation	Alpha
VAR (Variety)	1,7	5.76	2.14	.71
AUTON (Autonomy)	2,10	7.93	1.74	.49
INTER (Interpersonal interaction)	3,9	6.23	2.00	.37
TASKID (Task identity)	4,8	6.09	2.26	.60
FEED (Feedback)	5,11	4.64	1.97	.59
RESINT (Resident interaction)	6,12	6.16	2.28	.66

A check on the assumed dimensionality of these items was made by conducting a principal components analysis of all 12 items together. The (VARIMAX) rotated structure matrix is reported below with coefficients less than .4 omitted. As can be seen the *a priori* dimensions appear in a relatively straitforward manner. The two dimensions referring to the task integrity of the job (Variety and Task identity) combine in the first factor whilst Resident Interaction, Feedback and Autonomy separate into individual factors. The exception is Interpersonal interaction which shares variance with the first and second factors and obviously has less integrity as an independent measure.

Item number	Key	Factor 1	Factor 2	Factor 3	Factor 4
1	V	.64	—	—	—
2	A	—	—	—	.82
3	I	.65	—	—	—
4	T	.76	—	—	—
5	F	—	—	.69	—
6	R	—	.82	—	—
7	V	.64	.42	—	—
8	T	.72	—	—	—
9	I	—	.52	—	—
10	A	—	—	—	.63
11	F	—	—	.80	—
12	R	—	.74	—	—
Per cent explained variance		34.7	10.1	9.0	8.5

7. *Role Ambiguity and conflict*   The first six items of question 28 contribute to the scale of Role Ambiguity (AMBIG). These items were reverse scored from the values given in the questionnaire so that high scores represent greater ambiguity; the range is 6–42. The overall mean was 16.8, the standard deviation was 6.97 and Alpha = .84.

The next eight items of question 28 yield the scale for Role Conflict (CONF). Using the values as supplied in the questionnaire CONF has a range of 8–56. The overall mean was 31.5, standard deviation was 11.97 and Alpha = .84.

Whilst AMBIG was shown to consist of one factor by a principal components analysis, CONF yielded two factors. The first, explaining 48.2 per cent of the variance, linked items 7, 8, 9, 13 and 14 and the second, explaining 14.7 per cent of the variance, linked items 10, 11 and 12 which all refer to 'other people'. This seems to indicate role conflict having its origins in 'bureaucratic demands' (Factor 1) and 'interpersonal interactions' (Factor 2).

8. *Hierarchy of authority and participation*

The first five items of question 30 form the scale of perceived Hierarchy of authority (HIER). Scored as shown in the questionnaire HIER has a range of 5–25. The overall mean was 15.5, standard deviation was 5.33 and Alpha = .84.

The next four items of question 30 form a scale of perceived Participation in the organisation (PARTIC). These items were reverse-scored so that higher scores represent greater perceived participation. The overall mean was 12.95, standard deviation was 4.70 and Alpha = .84.

Both measures loaded on single factors in principal components analysis.

9. *Staff support*

Question 32 is comprised of three sections, each of two items, measuring support from supervisors (SUPSUP), fellow employees (PEERSUP) and subordinates (SUBSUP). Each item was scored 1–5 ('very little' = 1) so that each support scale has a range 2–10. The overall mean for SUPSUP was 7.28, standard deviation = 2.47, Alpha = .86; forPEERSUP the mean was 7.73, standard deviation = 1.93, Alpha = .83 and for SUBSUP the mean was 7.97, standard deviation = 1.18, Alpha = − 0.07. The pilot versions of these scales were much longer and predicted reliabilities for the two-item versions were high at .75. In the event SUPSUP and PEERSUP performed with higher reliability than this, but SUBSUP produced contradictory values and must be judged of little use as an additive scale. It was excluded from most multi-variate analyses in any case as it is only valid for those with formal authority (N = 89).

10. *Resident orientation*

Resident orientation (RESOR) focuses on attitudes to the residents as individuals and was measured by the eight items of question 33. These were scored 1–5 ('agree' = 1), with four items reverse-scored as shown in the reproduced questionnaire, so that higher scores indicate a tendency to agree with pro-normalisation values. The range is 8–40. The overall mean value was 32.71, standard deviation was 5.86 and Alpha = .77. A principal components analysis yielded one factor.

11. *Service orientation*

Service orientation (SERVOR) focuses on attitudes to the type of service provision for residents and was measured by the eight items of question

36. These were scored 1–5 ('agree' = 1), with four items reverse-scored as shown in the reproduced questionnaire, so that higher scores indicate a tendency to agree with pro-community service options. The range is 8–40. The overall mean value was 25.77, standard deviation was 6.57 and Alpha = .76. A principal components analysis yielded two factors; the first (39.4 per cent variance) grouped items 1, 2, 4 and 7 which are either pro-hospital or anti-community in sense; the second (23.2 per cent variance) grouped items 3, 5, 6 and 8 which are all pro-community. The second factor grouped the reverse-scored items. This analysis suggests that service options may be viewed as separate rather than opposite courses of action, but the result may also be an artifact of the scale design.

12. *Union attitudes*

Question 39 contains two sections: the first, of five items, measures perceived union effectiveness (UNEFFEC) and the second, of four items, measures perceived union legitimacy (UNLEGIT). Both scales were scored 1–5 ('disagree' or 'ineffective' = 1), which gives UNEFFEC a range of 5–25 and UNLEGIT a range of 4–20. The overall mean for UNEFFEC was 16.14, standard deviation was 4.35 and Alpha = .87. The mean for UNLEGIT was 16.67, standard deviation was 3.05 and Alpha = .78. Both scales loaded on single factors in a principal components analysis.

FIRST SOME QUESTIONS ABOUT YOUR EMPLOYMENT.

1. Please give your present work location. _____
   (e.g. Villa or ward No., house etc.)

2. What is your official job designation _____
   (e.g. N.A., Charge Nurse, etc.)

3. Are you on

Permanent night shift		or	Variable dayshift	

   (if other please
   give details) _____

4. Do you work

Full time		or	Part time	

   IF PART-TIME How many hours per week
   do you work _____

5. Do you ever work longer than your set hours

Yes	No

   IF YES How many hours overtime did you
   do during your last working week? (paid, or
   time off in lieu) _____

6. Do you ever contribute any voluntary
   (unpaid) hours of work?

Yes	No

   IF YES Approximately how many hours
   during your last working week? _____

7. Do you have a formal qualification relating
   to work with mentally handicapped people?

Yes	No

   IF YES What is it? _____

8. What other professional qualifications
   do you hold? _____

9. Have you had any in-service training during
   the last year?

Yes	No

   IF YES How many
   hours _____ or days _____

10. How satisfied were you with that training?

(tick one)

| | mean= | | s.d.= | | |
very satisfied	quite satisfied	unsure	not very satisfied	very dissatisfied	no training
3.94	0.40				

11. (Please answer this question even if you have not had any training) How much more training, if any, do you feel you might need to enable you to do the job effectively?

(tick one)

| mean= | | s.d.= | |
none	a bit more	quite a lot more	continuous up-dating
3.12	1.13		

12. How long have you worked in your present employment?

Number of months _____ or years _____

13. How long altogether have you had in jobs caring for mentally handicapped people?

Number of months _____ or years _____

14. What was your last job? (or other, e.g. housewife) _____

IF CONCERNED WITH CARING FOR MENTALLY HANDICAPPED PEOPLE

Was this job in a hospital ☐ or a community setting? ☐

Was this facility funded privately	voluntarily funded	or funded by the state

15. What was your main job before you began work with mentally handicapped people; or have you always worked with them?

IF THE SAME AS Q.14 PLEASE WRITE SAME _____

(Questions 16 and 17 combine to form Community Employment Orientation)

16. If for some reason you were to lose your job here, how likely is it that you would seek employment in a community-based service for mentally handicapped people?

(tick one)

| mean= | | s.d.= | |
Not very likely	unsure	quite likely	very likely
2.95	1.04	.43	

N=264

141

17. How concerned would you be if you had to take some other form of employment?

	mean=		s.d.=	
(tick one)	Not very concerned	unsure	quite concerned	very concerned
	2.59	1.1	.43	

18. Please write in the amount of your normal gross earnings, that is before deductions £   Is that per week; month; or year? (ring one)

NOW SOME PERSONAL DETAILS

19. How old are you (age last birthday)   years

20. Sex

Male	Female

21. What is your marital status?

(tick one)

Single	
Married or living as married	
Widowed	
Divorced or separated	

22. (IF APPLICABLE) What is your spouses'/partners' job (or last main job if presently not working?)

_____

23. How old were you when you left full-time education?   years

How many of these examinations have you passed?
(Write in the number passed or cross out if not relevant)

CSE	GCE O Level	GCE A Level	University Degree

24. Do you have any children aged under 16 who are living with you?

Yes	No

      IF YES How many

(These items comprise the Malaise measure)

25. Now, more generally, we would like to ask you about particular problems you may recently have had with your health:

PLEASE RING EITHER YES OR NO FOR EACH ITEM

		(Mean)
Do you often have backache?	Yes	No
		.29
Do you feel tired most of the time?	Yes	No
		.20
Do you often feel miserable or depressed?	Yes	No
		.15

Do you often have bad headaches?	Yes	.17	No
Do you often get worried about things?	Yes	.28	No
Do you usually have great difficulty in falling asleep or staying asleep?	Yes	.16	No
Do you usually wake unnecessarily early in the morning?	Yes	.23	No
Do you wear yourself out worrying about your health?	Yes	.02	No
Do you often get into a violent rage?	Yes	.03	No
Do people often annoy and irritate you?	Yes	.26	No
Have you at times had a twitching of the face, head or shoulders?	Yes	.06	No
Do you often suddenly become scared for no good reason?	Yes	.03	No
Are you scared to be alone when there are no friends near you?	Yes	.02	No
Are you easily upset or irritated?	Yes	.12	No
Are you frightened of going out alone or of meeting people?	Yes	.03	No
Are you constantly keyed up and jittery?	Yes	.03	No
Do you suffer from indigestion	Yes	.14	No
Do you often suffer from an upset stomach?	Yes	.10	No
Is your appetite poor?	Yes	.05	No
Does every little thing get on your nerves and wear you out?	Yes	.02	No
Does you heart often race like mad?	Yes	.07	No
Do you often have bad pains in your eyes?	Yes	.06	No
Are you troubled with rheumatism or fibrositis?	Yes	.13	No
Have you ever had a nervous breakdown?	Yes	.03	No

N=261

All the rest of the questions relate to aspects of your job. Question 26, for example, concerns your *feelings* about your work

26. How satisfied are you with the following aspects of your work?

mean=   s.d.=   item total=

	Very satisfied	Quite satisfied	Neither one nor the other	Quite dissat- isfied	Very dissat- isfied
Income	2.59	1.2	.34		
Job Security	2.96	1.3	.19		
Number of hours of work	4.11	.8	.36		
Flexibility of hours	3.95	.9	.38		
Ease of travel to work	3.64	1.3	.21		
Management and supervision by your superiors	3.26	1.2	.53		
Relationships with fellow workers	4.31	.8	.32		
Opportunities for advancement	2.88	1.1	.42		
Public respect for the sort of work you do	3.40	1.1	28		
Your own accomplishments	3.62	1.0	.52		
Developing your skills	3.28	1.1	.62		
Having challenges to meet	3.59	1.0	.62		
The actual tasks you do	3.70	1.0	.64		
The variety of tasks	3.60	1.1	.65		
Opportunities to use your own initiative	3.65	1.1	.62		
The physical work conditions	3.48	1.2	.44		
Your work in general	3.81	1.0	.60		

(PLEASE WRITE IN)   N=228

The one thing you like *best* about your job ———————————————

———————————————

The one thing you like *least* about your job ———————————————

———————————————

(These items provide the six Job Dimensions)

Questions 27 to 30 concern the *actual nature* of your job, rather than your feelings about it, so try to think how things really are at work when you answer them.

27.

	Very little (Key)	A little	A moderate amount	Quite a lot	A great deal
	key=	mean=	s.d.=	r with pair	N
How much variety is there in your job?	V	2.98	1.2	.55	257
How much are you left on your own to do your own work?	A	3.93	1.1	.32	257
To what extent is dealing with people other than residents a part of your job?	I	2.79	1.4	.23	257
How far do you see particular projects through to completion	T	2.82	1.4	.43	257
To what extent do you find out how well you are doing the job as you are working?	F	2.67	1.1	.42	257
How much opportunity is there for interaction with individual residents?	R	3.09	1.3	.49	257
What opportunities are there to do a number of different things in each working shift?	V	2.78	1.2	.55	
To what extent do your own activities contribute to the complete service provided for a resident?	T	3.27	1.3	.43	
How much opportunity is there to talk to other employees while at work?	I	3.44	1.1	.23	
To what extent are you able to act independently of supervision in performing your job?	A	4.0	1.1	.32	
How much information do you receive on your job performance?	F	1.97	1.1	.42	
How much of your job is directly concerned with interpersonal contact with residents, rather than other duties such as physical care?	R	3.08	1.3	.49	

KEY: V: Variety;   A: Autonomy;   I: Interpersonal Interaction;   T: Task Identity;
F: Feedback;   R: Resident Interaction

(The first six items of this question from the scale of 'Role Ambiguity', the rest comprise the scale of 'Role Conflict')

28. When answering this question, imagine a scale running from one to seven and tick the box that measures how much you think each statement applies to your job. Again, think about the *actual nature* of your job

	mean=	s.d.=	item total					
	Very false							Very true
	1	2	3	4	5	6	7	
I am certain about how much authority I have	2.86	1.7	.50					
Clear, planned goals and objectives exist for my job	3.79	1.8	.54					
I know that I have divided my time properly	3.09	1.6	.60					
I know what my responsibilities are	1.93	1.2	.60					
I know exactly what is expected of me	2.34	1.5	.66					
Explanation is clear of what has to be done	2.80	1.7	.65					
I have to do things that should be done differently	4.28	2.0	.55					
I receive an assignment without the staff to complete it	4.49	2.2	.66					
I have to bend or ignore a rule or policy in order to carry out an assignment	3.82	2.2	.61					
I work with two or more groups who operate quite differently	4.17	2.3	.43					
I receive incompatible requests from two or more people	3.40	2.1	.60					
I do things that are apt to be accepted by one person and not accepted by others	4.03	2.2	.63					
I receive an assignment without adequate resources to carry it out	4.28	2.2	.66					
I work on unnecessary things	3.03	2.1	.48					

N = 228

146

29. And more generally would you agree that:

Caring for the day-to-day needs of mentally handicapped people is more suitable work for women than men	2.31	2.1				
Among care staff men are more likely to be promoted than women	2.7	2.2				

(The first five items of this question comprise the scale of 'Hierarchy of Authority', the rest comprise 'Participation in Decisions')

30. Again imagine a scale from very false to very true and tick one box for each statement

mean =   s.d. =   item total

	Very false				Very true
	1	2	3	4	5
There can be little action taken here until someone in authority approves a decision	3.91	1.2	.60		
A person who wants to make his or her own decisions would be quickly discouraged	2.79	1.3	.49		
Even small matters have to be referred to someone higher-up for a final answer	3.31	1.5	.73		
I have to ask my immediate supervisor before I do almost anything	2.46	1.4	.72		
Any decision I make has to have my superior's approval	3.03	1.4	.70		
Participation in decisions is very limited	3.15	1.4	.61		
Consultation about changes is rare	2.92	1.5	.60		
I feel I have no say in the day-to-day running of this place	3.35	1.5	.70		
My opinion does not count when a problem comes up	3.54	1.3	.77		

N = 248

(The two parts of question 31 form the scale 'Propensity to Leave')

31. How likely is it that you will actively look for a new job next year?

mean =   s.d. =   curr with pair

Extremely unlikely	Quite unlikely	Unsure, maybe	Quite likely	Extremely likely
2.89	1.53	.64		

N = 261

Do you think about leaving your job ......?

Never	Rarely	Sometimes	Rather often	Nearly all the time
2.85	1.14	.64		

(Support measures)

32.   Thinking now about the various people with whom you work:

Concerning your immediate superior

mean =   s.d. =   curr with
pair =

please estimate:–	Very little	Little	A mode-rate amount	Quite a lot	A great deal
How much he/she is willing to listen to your problems	3.71	1.25	.77		
How much you can trust him/her	3.57	1.38	.77		

N = 261

Concerning your work group/fellow employees

please estimate:–	Very little	Little	A mode-rate amount	Quite a lot	A great deal
How well they work together and offer each other support	3.89	1.03	.71		
How willing they are to listen to your problems	3.83	1.06	.71		

N = 260

THIS PART OF QUESTION 32 IS TO BE ANSWERED ONLY BY THOSE WITH FORMAL AUTHORITY (eg Sisters/charge nurses, etc: including those 'acting up')

Concerning your subordinates

please estimate:–	Very little	Little	A mode-rate amount	Quite a lot	A great deal
How much work they expect of you	4.0	.78	−.03		
How friendly and easy to approach they are	4.0	.91	−.03		

N = 89

(Question 33 gives the 'Resident Orientation')

The next set of questions asks about your knowledge and opinions on aspects of your work.

33.

	mean =	s.d. =	item total		
Thinking about what you know of residents:	Agree	Tend to agree	Uncertain	Tend to disagree	Disagree
Mentally handicapped residents appreciate attractive surroundings	4.27	.9	.46	R*	
Therapy can achieve little with severely handicapped residents	3.88	1.3	.63		
Sexually active residents should be sterilised	3.40	1.5	.42		
Residents can respond to care	4.81	.4	.48	R	
Residents should not be treated like young children	4.30	1.1	.36	R	
Most residents will never know right from wrong	3.75	1.3	.53		
Little can be done to help severely handicapped residents to improve	4.05	1.2	.69		
Residents can often lead a life which is just as valuable as anyone else's	4.25	1.2	.42	R	

N = 255

34. Thinking about your unit (ward, villa, house, etc) as a whole can you please estimate the AVERAGE level of dependency of your residents. Are they mostly:—

Low dependency	Medium dependency	High dependency
2.38	0.66	

TICK ONLY ONE BOX.

*Item reversed scored.

149

35. What proportion of the residents on your unit have severe behaviour problems?

None	Very few	Quite a few	About half	Quite a lot	Most	All
3.2	1.60					

TICK ONE BOX.

(Question 36 gives the 'Service Orientation')

36.

	mean =	s.d. =	item total		
Thinking about the type of service:	Agree	Tend to agree	Uncertain	Tend to disagree	Disagree
It is inevitable that mentally handicapped people will not be properly cared for in the community	3.13	1.3	.48		
Mentally handicapped people are safer in hospital	2.44	1.5	.59		
Only a community based home or hostel can provide the sort of life that mentally handicapped people should have	3.02	1.4	.23	R*	
There will never be the right facilities for mentally handicapped people in the community	2.86	1.3	.41		
Residents will respond to care much more readily in a community home of hostel	3.35	1.3	.41	R	
Some kind of community service will always be preferable for the mentally handicapped person compared to being a resident in a hospital	3.50	1.3	.64	R	
Specialised hospitals are the best places for mentally handicapped people	3.34	1.4	.60		
Small community units are bound to be run more effectively than large hospitals	3.62	1.3	.35	R	

N = 253

*Item reversed scored.

37. How likely do you think it is that the following things will happen.

	Very unlikely	Not likely	Unsure	Quite likely	Very likely
That not all mentally handicapped people will be discharged into the community	3.64	1.39			
That the 'move to the community' will produce a poor service	3.32	1.13			
That the public will accept mentally handicapped people in the community	2.45	1.17			

38. Are you a member of a trade union or professional association?

Yes	No

IF YES Which is it? ....

(Question 39 gives the 'Union Effectiveness' in the first five items and 'Union Legitimacy' in the final four items)

39. Please answer this question even if you are not a member of a union or professional association and, in the first part, think about what you know of unions at work).

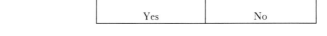

mean =   s.d. =   item total

To what extent do you think your local union is effective in ...	Very effective	Rather effective	Unsure	Quite effective	Very effective
Improving pay and working conditions	2.78	1.1	.60		
Protecting individuals from favouritism or persecution	3.36	1.1	.71		
Ensuring fair treatment of employees	3.52	1.1	.78		
Protecting the staff's interests in cases of controversy	3.58	1.0	.75		
Participating in the business of decision making	2.90	1.1	.66		

N = 256

Thinking about unions more generally, do you agree that ...	Disagree	Tend to disagree	Not sure	Tend to agree	Agree
Staff working as we do need the protection of a union	4.47	.83	.65		
More staff should be members of a union	4.08	1.1	.66		
Unions are useful in the conduct of industrial relations	4.25	.88	.60		
It is quite right that unions should have a say in the running of our service	3.87	1.1	.48		

N = 256

40. In this question please estimate how much effect you think each level of authority has on the situation. For each statement below give what you think is the order of importance of each level by WRITING IN the numbers 1 to 4, as we have shown in the example of 'setting pay levels'.

DO NOT USE TICKS IN THESE BOXES.

How much effect does each level of authority have on:—	Local management	District	Region	Government
(e.g. only) setting pay levels	4	3	1	2
Producing general uncertainty				
Creating problems for the provision of effective care				
Bringing about low morale				
Making policy that directly affects you in your job				
Causing confusion amongst staff				

PLEASE CHECK THROUGH TO BE SURE YOU HAVE ANSWERED ALL THE QUESTIONS. THANK YOU.

If there are any problems relating to your job or this questionnaire which you would like to bring to our attention, please write about them here. You can write on the back of these sheets, if necessary.

1. Comments on postal interview and research

2. Work location and resident characteristics (nursing, physical, behaviour, sex, staffing level)

3. Length of service

4. Previous service (hospital name, type of other work experience)

5. Qualifications

6. Marital status; dependents; earning status (check sharing of income)

7. Area of residence (check willingness to move)

8. Reasons for joining employment (check knowledge of job; first contact)

9. Contacts with MH and the job
(a) Prior knowledge (relatives eg)
(b) Friends working

10. Status of work: how thought seen by friends etc.

11. Motivation
(a) Very much personally involved in the work?
(b) Extent to which that involvement is approved
(c) Do voluntary work? (elsewhere?)
(d) Is the job a major part of your identity?

12. Intentions
(a) Specific job intentions (career progression)
(b) More general ambitions (5 years time?)
(c) Specific implications of closure

13. Leaving: if you leave here would it be–
(a) To get away from job (stress, other people)
(b) To improve (or part of a plan)
(c) To avoid closure problems
(d) Just to change

14. Expectations:
(a) Is the job what you expected (check source of prior info)
(b) How do you feel about match between conditions and expectations
(c) Can situation change
(d) How did you adapt

L

15. Training:

(a) Give details (titles, length, content, appraisal)
(b) Present requirements (identify specific problems)
(c) Nature of training thought best
(d) Relationship to experience (useful in community?)
(e) Relevance to changing situation (check new syllabus)
(f) Do trained staff differ? (how)

16. Job:

(a) What do you do? (typical day, estimate time periods)
(b) How does this contribute to Variety? (Task identity)
(c) Examples of Autonomy (decisions)

  (i)   Buying in (eg linen) who does decide
  (ii)   Getting repairs done who does decide
  (iii) Residents' holidays who does decide
  (iv)   Individual programmes who does decide
  (v)   Staff rota/shift who does decide

(d) Who interact with; in what ways (Inter)
(e) How and when interact with residents (Resint)
(f) Feedback: how; from whom; how often; what sort (eg on job performance) (identify specific lacks)

17. Values:

(a) Describe work role (terms: nurse, carer, teacher, domestic, servant)
(b) What should service be like ideally (specifics)
(c) How far should 'normalisation' go (hire staff, instruct staff)
(d) Are policies right? (what needs doing; correcting)

18. Organisations:

(a) How much do you need to know about system to operate
(b) Identify problems in the organisation of work (hierarchy)
(c) Who is responsible for these problems
(d) Problems with other services (eg GPs)

19. Conditions:

(a) Unions: why join; how useful
(b) What *are* conditions of service

  (i)   structure of career/salary
  (ii)   pensions/status
  (iii) progression (gender)

20. Support:

(a) Who gives (emotional) support (gender)
(b) How often possible (include phone)
(c) Time available (separate formal/informal)
(d) Do superiors actively seek to provide support
(e) Do supporters circumvent hierarchy (and be positive)

(f)   Quality of decision-type support (back-up for autonomy)

(g)   Specific needs/suggestion

(h)   Identify any support lacks connected with closure (eg constraints on time, management contact)

21.   Satisfaction: (Community: VAR; AUTON; role AMBIG; HIER) or (Hospital: FEED; RESINT; AMBIG; CONF, DEPEN, INTER)

(a)   How do you feel you are affected by (as above)

(b)   How cope (or otherwise respond)

(c)   Give specific examples of problems

(d)   How does job performance relate to these

22.   Stress: (Community: AUTON: PARTIC; AMBIG;) or (Hospital: RESINT, TASKID)

(a)   are there especially stressful things (list them)

(b)   how handle these (how improve on coping)

(c)   What organisation ('Management' and/or 'System') factors contribute most to your feelings (of stress)

(d)   What factors associated with closure do?

Appendix 2

Abbreviations used in the text

CN/S	Charge Nurse/Sister
CoHSE	Confederation of Health Service Employees
CSS	Certificate in Social Services
(S)EN(MH)	(Senior) Enrolled Nurse (Mental Handicap)
ICP	Individual Care Plan
MSC	Manpower Services Commission
NA	Nursing Assistant
NALGO	National Association of Local Government Officers
NHS	National Health Service
NO	Nursing Officer
NUPE	National Union of Public Employees
PCSC	Preliminary Certificate in Social Care
RCN	Royal College of Nursing
RHA	Regional Health Authority
RN(MH)	Registered Nurse (Mental Handicap)
RNMS	Registered Nurse for the Mentally Subnormal

References

Alaszewski, A (1986) *Institutional Care and the Mentally Handicapped*, Croom Helm, London

Allen, P (1983) Training direct care staff. In: Ann Shearer (ed) *An Ordinary Life*, Project Paper 42, Kings Fund, London

Aiken, M and Hage, T (1966) Organisational alienation: a comparative analysis, *American Sociological Review*, *31*, 497–507

Anderson, D (1982) *Social Work and Mental Handicap*, Macmillan/BASW, London

Bartol, K M (1979) Professionalism as a predictor of organisational commitment, role stress, and turnover: a multi-dimensional approach, *Academy of Management Journal*, *22*, 815–821

Baysinger, B D and Mobley, W H (1983) Employee turnover: individual and organisational analysis. In: *Research in Personnel and Human Resources Management*, J A I Press, Greenwich, Conn.

Bebbington, A C and Quine, L (1987) A comment on Hirst's 'Evaluating the malaise inventory', *Social Psychiatry*, *22*, 5–7

Benton, D A and White, C H (1972) Satisfaction with job factors for registered nurses, *Journal of Nursing Administration*, December, 55–63

Bjaanes, A T and Butler, E W (1974) Environmental variation in community care facilities for mentally retarded persons, *American Journal of Mental Deficiency*, *78*, 429–439

Bradshaw, J, Cooke, K, Glendinning, C, Baldwin, S, Lawton, D and Staden, F (1982) *1970 Cohort: 10 year Follow-up Study*, Interim Report to the DHSS 108/6.82

Brief, A P and Aldag, R J (1976) Correlates of role indices, *Journal of Applied Psychology*, *61*, 468–472

Brief, A P and Aldag, R J (1978) The job characteristics inventory: an examination, *Academy of Management Journal*, *21*, 659–670

Briggs Committee (1972) *Report of the Committee on Nursing*, Cmnd. 5115, HMSO, London

Brown, J and Walton, I (1984) *How Nurses Learn: A National Study of the Training of Nurses in Mental Handicap*, University of York

Bryant, D J (1965) A survey of the development of manpower planning policies, *British Journal of Industrial Relations*, *3*, 279–290

Caplan, R D (1971) *Organisational Stress and Individual Strain: A Social Psychological Study of Risk Factors in Coronary Heart Disease Among Administrators, Engineers and Scientists*. Institute for Social Research, University of Michigan, Microfilm 72–14822, Ann Arbor, Michigan

Carr, J (1985) The effect of the severely abnormal on their families. In: A M Clarke and A D B Clarke (eds) *Mental Deficiency: The Changing Outlook*, Methuen, London

Cartwright, L K (1979) Sources of and effects of stress in health careers. In: G C Stone and N E Adler (eds) *Health Psychology*, Jossey Bas, San Francisco

CCETSW (1986) *Staff Development in the Field of Mental Handicap*. Summary of Conferences at Harrogate and Birmingham, CCETSW, London

Cooper, C and Payne, R (eds) (1978) *Stress at Work*, Wiley, London

Corwin, R (1961) The professional employee: a study of conflict in nursing roles. *American Journal of Sociology*, *66*, 604–615

Daniel, W W (1971) Industrial behaviour and the orientation to work: a critique, *Journal of Management Studies*, *8*, 329–335

Davies, C (1983) Professionals in bureaucracies: the conflict thesis revisited. In: Robert Dingwell and Philip Lewis (eds) *The Sociology of the Professions*, Macmillan, London

Davies, C and Rosser, J (1986) *Processes of Discrimination: report on a study of women working in the NHS*, DHSS, London

Davis, L E and Cherns, A B (1975) *The Quality of Working Life*, Vol. 1, The Free Press, Macmillan, New York

Decker, F H (1985) Socialisation and interpersonal environment in nurses' affective reactions to work, *Social Science and Medicine*, *20*, 5, 499–509

DHSS (1969) *Report of the Committee of Inquiry into Allegations of Ill-treatment of Patients and Other Irregularities at the Ely Hospital, Cardiff*, HMSO, London

DHSS (1971) *Better Services for the Mentally Handicapped*, Cmnd. 4683, HMSO, London

DHSS (1980) *Mental Handicap: Progress, Problems and Priorities*, HMSO, London

DHSS (1983) *Health Service Development: Care in the Community and Joint Finance*, HC (83/6)

DHSS (1974 to 1987) *Health and Personal Social Services Statistics for England*, HMSO, London

DHSS (1985) *Government Response to the Second Report from the Social Services Committee 1984–5 session. Community Care: with special reference to adult mentally ill and mentally handicapped people*. Cmnd. 9674, HMSO, London

Dingwall, R W J (1972) Nursing: towards a male dominated occupation? *Nursing Times, 68*, 1294–1295

Dingwall, R and McIntosh, J (1978) *Readings in the Sociology of Nursing*, Churchill Livingstone, London

Dingwall, R and Lewis, P (1983) *The Sociology of the Professions*, Macmillan, London

East Anglian Regional Health Authority, *Regional Strategic Plan 1984–85 to 1993–94*, 46–61, EARHA, Cambridge

Elliott, P (1972) *The Sociology of the Professions*, Macmillan, London

English National Board (1982) *Syllabus of Training: Professional Register*, part 5 (Registered Nurse for the Mentally Handicapped) ENB, London

Evans, G, Todd, S and Blunden, R (1984) *Working in a comprehensive community based service for mentally handicapped people: a survey of the staff of the NIMROD service*, Mental Handicap in Wales, Applied Research Unit, Cardiff

Felce, D (1983) Selection, recruitment and promotion. In: Ann Shearer (ed) *An Ordinary Life*, Project Paper 42, Kings Fund, London

Fusilier, M R, Ganster, D, and Mayes, B T (1986) The social support and health relationship: and is there a gender difference? *Journal of Occupational Psychology, 59*, 145–153

George, L K (1983) Nursing turnover in long-term care institutions. In: I Simpson and R Simpson (eds) *Research in the Sociology of Work*, JAI Press, London

Ghiselli, E E, Campbell, J P and Zedeck, S (1981) *Measurement Theory for Behavioural Sciences*, W H Freeman and Co. San Francisco

Glick, W, Mirvis, P and Harder, D (1977) Union satisfaction and participation, *Industrial Relations, 16*, 145–151

GNCs/CCETSW (1982) *Co-operation in Training, Part 1 – Qualifying Training. Report of the Joint Working Group on Training for Staff Working with Mentally Handicapped People*, GNCs/CCETSW

Goffman, E (1964) *Stigma: notes on the management of spoiled identity*, Penguin Harmondsworth

Gray-Toft, P and Anderson, J G (1981) Stress among hospital nursing staff: its causes and effects, *Social Science and Medicine, 15A*, 639–647

Gray-Toft, P A and Anderson, J G (1985) Organisational stress in the hospital: development of a model for diagnosis and prediction, *Health Services Research, 19*, 6, Part 1, 753–774

Greenhaus, J H (1971) Self-esteem as an influence on occupational choice and occupational satisfaction, *Journal of Vocational Behaviour, 1*, 75–83

Griffiths Report (1983) *NHS Management Inquiry*, DHSS, London

Griffiths, Sir Roy (1988) Community care: agenda for action. Report to the Secretary of State for Social Services, HMSO, London

Gupta, N and Beehr, T A (1979) Job stress and employees' behaviour, *Organisational behaviour and Human Performance, 23*, 373–387

Hage, J and Aiken, M (1967) Relationship of centralisation to other structural properties, *Administrative Science Quarterly, 12*, 72–92

Hampson, R, Judge, K and Renshaw, J (1984) *Care in the Community*, Discussion paper 362/2, Personal Social Services Research Unit, University of Kent

Harris, A (1963) *Labour Mobility in Britain*, HMSO, London

Herzberg, F, Mausner, B and Snyderman, B (1959) *The Motivation to Work*, Wiley, New York

Hickson, D J, Hinings, C R, Lee, C A, Schneck, R E and Pennings, J M (1971) A strategic contingencies theory of intraorganisational power. *Administrative Science Quarterly, 16*, 216–229

Hockey, L (1976) *Women in Nursing*, Hodder and Stoughton, London

Holland, T (1973) Organisational structure and institutional care, *Journal of Health and Social Behaviour, 14*, 241–251

House of Commons (1985–6) *Government Response to the Second Report from the Social Services Committee, 1984–5 Session. Community Care – with special reference to adult mentally ill and mentally handicapped people. Vols. I–III*, HMSO, London

Ivancevich, J M and Matteson, M T (1981) *Stress at Work*, Scott, Foresman, Glenview, Illinois

Jabes, J (1978) *Individual Processes in Organisational Behaviour*, AHM, Illinois

Jamal, M (1984) Job stress and job performance controversy: an empirical assessment, *Organisational Behaviour and Human Performance, 33, 1–21*

Janicki, M P, Jacobson, J W, Zigman, W B and Gordon, N H (1984) Characteristics of employees of community residences for retarded persons, *Education and Training of the Mentally Retarded, 19*, 45–48

Jay Committee (1979) *Report of the Committee of Enquiry into Mental Handicap Nursing and Care*. Vol. I and II, Cmnd. 7468–1, 7468–II, HMSO, London

Johnson, T W and Stinson, J E (1975) Role ambiguity, role conflict and satisfaction: moderating effects of individual differences, *Journal of Applied Psychology, 60*, 329–333

Jones, E E and Nisbett, R E (1971) *The Actor and the Observer: divergent perceptions of the causes of behaviour*. General Learning Press, New York

Jones, K (1975) *Opening the Door*, Routledge and Kegan Paul, London

Jones, K and Fowles, A J (1984) *Ideas on Institutions: analysing the literature on long term care and custody*. Routledge, London

Kahn, R L, Wolfe, D M, Quinn, R P, Snock, J D and Rosenthal, R (1964) *Organisational Stress: Studies in Role Conflict and Ambiguity*. Wiley, New York

Katz, D and Kahn, R L (1966) *The Social Psychology of Organisations* 2nd. ed. (1978) Wiley, New York

Kenney, J, Donnelly, E and Reid, M (1979) *Manpower Training and Development* I P M, London

King, R, Raynes N and Tizard, J (1971) *Patterns of Residential Care: Sociological Studies in Institutions for Handicapped Children.* Routledge and Kegan Paul, London

King's Fund (1980) reprinted (1982) *An Ordinary Life: Comprehensive Locally-based Residential Services for Mentally Handicapped People.* Project Paper 24, Kings Fund Centre, London

Knapp, M, Harisis, K and Missiakoulis, S (1981) Who leaves social work. *British Journal of Social Work, 11,* 421–444

Knapp, M. Harisis, K and Missiakoulis, S (1982) Investigating labour turnover and wastage using the logit technique. *Journal of Occupational Psychology, 55,* 129–138

Korman, N and Glennerster, H (1984) The Darenth Park Project: a narrative of hospital closure. LSE, London. Now published as *Closing a Hospital,* Bedford Square Press, London

Kruglanski, A W (1970) Attributing trustworthiness in supervisor-worker relations. *Journal of Experimental Social Psychology, 6,* 214–232

Lyons, T F (1971) Role clarity, need for clarity, satisfaction, tension and withdrawal. *Organisational Behaviour and Human Performance, 6,* 99–110

Malin, N (1987) Community Care: Principles, Policy and Practice. Ch. 1 in *Reassessing Community Care,* Croom Helm, London

Malin, N, Race, D and Jones, G (1980) *Services for the Mentally Handicapped in Britain,* Croom Helm, London

Manpower Services Commission (1984) *Employers' Recruitment Practices,* MSC Gazette, Special Feature, pp.5–6

Mansell, J, Felce, D, Jenkins, J, De Kock, U, Toogood, S (1987) *Developing Staffed Housing for People with Mental Handicaps,* Costello, Tunbridge Wells

March, J G and Simon, H A (1958) *Organisations,* Wiley, New York

Matz, F (1969) Nurses. In A Etzioni (ed) *The Semi-Professions and their Organisation.* Free Press, Glencoe

McLain, R E, Silverstein, A B, Hubbell, M and Brownlee, L (1975) The characterisation of residential environments within a hospital for the mentally retarded. *Mental Retardation, 13,* 24–27

Mercer, G M (1979) *The Employment of Nurses: Nursing Labour Turnover in the NHS,* Croom Helm, London

Mersey Regional Health Authority (1985) *Regional Strategy 1985–1994,* 33–36, MRHA, Liverpool

Miles, R H (1975) An empirical test of causal inference between role perception of conflict and ambiguity and various personal outcomes. *Journal of Applied Psychology, 60*, 334–339

Miller, H E, Katerberg, C H and Hulin, C H (1979) Evaluation of the Mobley, Horner and Hollingsworth model of employee turnover. *Journal of Applied Psychology, 64*, 509–517

Moores, B and Grant, G (1977) Optimists and pessimists: attitudes of nursing staff towards the development potential of mentally handicapped patients in their charge. *International Journal of Nursing Studies, 14*, 13–18

Morris, P (1969) *Put Away: a Sociological Study of Institutions for the Mentally Retarded*, Routledge and Kegan Paul, London

National Union of Public Employees and the Low Pay Unit (1987) *Nursing a Grievance: Low Pay in Nursing*, NUPE and LPU, London

Nnadozie, J and Eldar, R (1985) Preference of hospital employees for work-related outcomes. *Social Science and Medicine, 21*, 6, 651–653

North East Thames Regional Health Authority (1984) *Regional Strategic Plan, 1984–1993*, 113–123, NETRHA, London

Northern Regional Health Authority (1986) *Regional Strategic Plan 1985–1994*, 85–102, NRHA, Newcastle upon Tyne

Northern West Thames Regional Health Authority (1985) *Regional Strategic Framework for 1994*, 25–27, NWTRHA, London

North Western Regional Health Authority (1985) *Regional Strategic Plan 1983–1993*, 168–173, NWRHA, Manchester

Oxford Regional Health Authority (1984) *Regional Strategic Plan 1984–1994*, 375–282, ORHA, Oxford

Pahl, J and Quine, L (1985) *Families with Mentally Handicapped Children: a study of stress and of service response*. Health Services Research Unit, University of Kent

Pahl, J and Roose, G (1990) *Training Staff to Work in Community Care Services*, Centre for Health Services Studies, University of Kent

Peat, Marwick (1986) *Current Issues in Public Sector Management*, Peat, Marwick, Mitchel and Co. London

Pettman, B (1973) Some factors influencing labour turnover: a review of research literature. *Industrial Relations, 4*, 43–61

Pierce, J L and Dunham, R B (1978) An empirical demonstration of the convergence of common macro- and micro-organisational measures. *Academy of Management Journal, 21*, 410–418

Pierce, J L, Dunham, R B and Blackburn, R S (1979) Social systems structure, job design, and growth need strength: a test of a congruency model. *Academy of Management Journal, 22*, 223–240

Plank, M (1982) *Teams for Mentally Handicapped People*, CMH, London

Pratt, M W, Luszcz, M A and Brown, M E (1980) Measuring dimensions of the quality of care in small community residences. *American Journal of Mental Deficiency, 85,* 188–194

Price, J (1977) *The Study of Turnover,* Iowa State University Press

Quine, L (1986) Behaviour problems in severely mentally handicapped children. *Psychological Medicine, 16,* 895–907

Radford, N H (1985) *Strategies for Change: Training in Mental Handicap Nursing,* University of Surrey

Radford, N H (1988) Be prepared. *Nursing Times,* January 6–12, p.66

Rawlings, S A (1985) Life-styles of severely retarded non-communicating adults in hospitals and small residential homes. *British Journal of Social Work, 15,* 281–293

Raynes, N V, Pratt, M W and Roses, S (1979) *Organisational Structure and the Care of the Mentally Retarded.* Croom Helm, London

Redfern, S J and Spurgeon, S (1980) Hospital sisters: work attitudes, perceptions and wastage. *Journal of Advanced Nursing, 5,* 5, 451–466

Rizzo, J, House, R J and Lirtzman, S I (1970) Role conflict and ambiguity in complex organisations. *Administrative Science Quarterly, 15,* 150–163

Royal College of Nursing (1987) *Face the Facts on Nursing,* RCN, London

Rutter, M, Tizard, J and Whitmore, K (1970a) *Education, Health and Behaviour,* Longmans, London

Rutter, M, Graham, P and Yule, W (1970b) *A Neuropsychiatric Study in Childhood,* Heinemann, London

Rutter, M, Yule, B, Quinton, D, Towland, O, Yule, W and Berger, M (1975) Attainment and adjustment in two geographical areas. *British Journal of Psychiatry, 126,* 520–523

Saunders, C (1981) *Social Stigma of Occupations,* Gower, Farnborough

Schuler, R S, Aldag, R J and Brief, A P (1977) Role conflict and ambiguity: a scale analysis. *Organisational Behaviour and Human Performance, 20,* 111–128

Seashore, S E, Lawler, E E, Mirvis, P and Cammann, C (eds) (1982) *Observing and Measuring Organisational Change: a guide to field practice.* Wiley, New York

Secretaries of State for Health (1989) *Caring for People: Community Care in the Next Decade and Beyond,* Cm 849, HMSO, London

Seybolt, J W and Pavett, C M (1979) The prediction of effort and performance among hospital professionals: moderating effects of feedback on expectancy theory formulations. *Journal of Occupational Psychology, 52,* 91–105

Sheridan, J E and Vredenburgh, D J (1978) Usefulness of leadership behaviour and social power variables in predicting job tension, performance, and turnover of nursing employees. *Journal of Applied Psychology, 63,* 1, 89–95

Sims, H P, Szilagyi, A D and Keller, R T (1976) The measurement of job characteristics. *Academy of Management Journal, 19*, 195–212

South East Thames Regional Health Authority (1986) *Regional Strategic Plan, 1985–1994*, 83–105, SETRHA, Bexhill-on-Sea

South West Thames Regional Health Authority (1985) *Regional Strategic Plan 1985–94*, Section 22, SWTRHA, London

South Western Regional Health Authority (1985) *Regional Strategy 1985–94*, 21–27, SWRHA, Bristol

St Claire, L (1986) Mental retardation: impairment or handicap? *Disability, Handicap and Society, 1*, 233–243

Steers, R M and Mowday, R T (1980) Employee turnover and post-decision accommodation processes. *In C C Cummings and B M Staw (eds) Research in Organisational Behaviour*, JAI Press, Greenwich

Strauss, A L, Schatzman, C, Bucher, R, Ehrlich, D and Subshin, M (1964) *Psychiatric Ideologies and Institutions*, Free Press, New York

Strickland, L H (1958) Surveillance and trust. *Journal of Personality, 28*, 200–215

Szilagyi, A D (1977) An empirical test of causal inference between role perceptions, satisfaction with work, performance and organisational level. *Personnel Psychology, 30*, 375–388

Szilagyi, A D, Sims, H P and Keller, R T (1976) Role dynamics, locus of control, and employee attitudes and behaviour. *Academy of Management Journal, 19*, 259–276

Taylor, J and Taylor, D (1986) *Mental handicap: partnership in the community.* Office of Health Economics/Mencap, London

Thompson, J (1967) *Organisations in Action*, McGraw Hill, New York

Tizard, J (1964) *Community Services for the Mentally Handicapped*, Oxford University Press, Oxford

Tizard, J, Sinclair, I and Clarke, R V G (1975) *Varieties of Residential Experience*, Routledge and Kegan Paul, London

Torgerson, W S (1958) *Theory and Methods of Scaling*, Wiley, New York

Trent Regional Health Authority (1986) *Better Health for Trent – a plan for action, 1983/84–1993/94*, TRHA, Sheffield

Tyne, A and O'Brien J (1981) *The Principle of Normalisation: a foundation for effective services*, CMH, London

United Nations General Assembly (1972) *Declaration on the Rights of Mentally Retarded Persons*, Resolution 2856, 26th Session, para 88

Uphoff, W H and Dunnette, M D (1956) *Understanding the Union Member*, University of Minnesota, Minneapolis

Wanous, J P (1980) *Organisational Entry*, Addison-Wesley, Reading, Mass.

Ward, L (1984) *Planning for People: Developing a Local Service for People with Mental Handicap*, Kings Fund, London

Ward, L (1985) Training staff for 'an ordinary life'. Experiences in a community service in South Bristol. *British Journal of Mental Subnormality, 32*, Part 2, 94–102

Weiner, Y and Vardi, Y (1980) Relationship between job, organisation and career commitments and work outcomes: an integrative approach. *Organisational Behaviour and Human Performance, 26*, 81–96

Wertheimer, A (1986) *Hospital Closures in the Eighties*, Campaign for People with Mental Handicaps, London

West Midlands Regional Health Authority (1985) *A Strategy for Health 1984–1994, Vol. II*, Individual Service Reviews, 38–55. WMRHA, Birmingham

Wolfensberger, W (1972) *The Principle of Normalisation in Human Services.* National Institute on Mental Retardation, Toronto

Wolfensberger, W (1980) The definition of normalisation: update, problems, disagreements and misunderstandings. In: R J Flynn and K E Nitsch (eds) *Normalisation, Social Integration and Community Services*, University Park Press, Baltimore

Wolfensberger, W and Glenn, L (1975) *Program Analysis of Service Systems (PASS)*, National Institute on Mental Retardation, Toronto

Wolfensberger, W and Thomas, S (1983) *PASSING: Programme Analysis of Service Systems Implementation of Normalisation Goals*, National Institute on Mental Retardation, Toronto

Yorkshire Regional Health Authority (1987) *Strategic Plan 1985/86–1993/94*, 34–36, YRHA, Harrogate

Zigman, W B, Schwartz, A A and Janicki, M P (1982) *Group Home Employee Job Attitudes and Satisfactions*, LARP, New York State Institute for Basic Research, New York.

Printed by HMSO, Edinburgh Press
Dd 0292953 3M 6/90 (279446)